Praise for *Greener Cleaner*

"As you read Dr. Sneller's book you can't help but be impressed by his in-depth coverage of so many aspects of your health in relation to your everyday exposures. This book succinctly covers what you want and need to know to protect yourself and your loved ones. This book may save your life."

Doris J. Rapp, MD, Pediatrician,
Allergist and Environmental Medical Specialist

"Dr. Sneller's explanation of airline travel is an accurate depiction of our flying experience today. As a pilot for many years, I can testify that it is important for those of us in the industry to keep the public abreast of changes that directly affect them, hence my support for his chapter on Traveling by Commercial Airplane in *Greener Cleaner Indoor Air*.

Steve Pierce, Captain, 26 years

"As a parent, I find *Greener Cleaner Indoor Air* an outstanding reference manual. It not only serves as a guide for me to understand my allergies and behavior, but offers a great deal of knowledge for my own betterment. I have found this book to be an invaluable addition to my library. It is educational and original.

Lynn Wiese Sneyd, author of Holistic Parenting: Raising Children to a New Physical, Emotional, and Spiritual Well-Being

"Dr. Sneller's review of nasal allergy and asthma in *Greener Cleaner Indoor Air: A Guide to Healthier Living* presents a large volume of important material. Generally, the facts are presented in a clear manner and understandable to the reader. As the author suggests, those with symptoms that impair quality of life should seek medical consultation and treatment.

Gerald Goldstein, MD, Diplomate of the American Board of Allergy and Clinical Immunology

Greener Cleaner Indoor Air

Greener Cleaner Indoor Air

A Guide to Healthier Living

Mark R. Sneller

Greener Cleaner Indoor Air: A Guide to Healthier Living

Published by Wheatmark®
610 East Delano Street, Suite 104
Tucson, Arizona 85705 U.S.A.
www.wheatmark.com

International Standard Book Number: 978-1-60494-234-7
Library of Congress Control Number: 2009928154

This book is dedicated to my mother, who gave me my first books to read and taught me to persevere.

I once told her that I would be an old man by the time I got out of school. She replied, "You're going to be an old man anyway, so you might as well be a smart old man."

Did You Know

- The refrigerator in the kitchen is the worst area of the home to harbor bacteria, mold, and viruses both inside and outside, and the laundry room may be the second worst room of the home?

- Painful arthritis and headaches occur when the barometric pressure drops and storms are coming in?

- Most homes that have cat antigen present never had a cat?

- No major medical organization subscribes to the concept that there is toxic mold that affects our health through inhalation?

- Most homes have numerous pesticides in the air and furnishings—pesticides that were never used?

- Four simple and inexpensive cleaning agents can save you hundreds of dollars a year, lessen your trips to the doctor, and give you, your children and pets a healthier environment?

- The EPA classifies fragrances and perfumes as hazardous?

- Ozone machines and air purifiers have never been found to be clinically effective?

- There is no asbestos problem in our nation's schools?

- Only under the rarest of circumstances is asbestos a problem for the home owner?

- Everyday chemicals affect our children's ability to learn?

- Pollen antigens can affect us even when it is off season?

- Food and pollen can have similar antigens?

- Household dust is comprised of over fifty different particle types?

- Dust and pesticides enter the home most frequently through tracking and that taking off the shoes at the door can reduce the dust level significantly?

- The appearance of a home can be deceiving and when buying one, the local plants and traffic must be taken into consideration?

- Fifty percent of all Americans who have allergies are allergic to cats?

- Asthma is on the increase?

- We are ten times as likely to get cancer from our indoor environment than from outdoors?

- Many art supplies are now non toxic?

- Indoors there are more emissions from paint than from carpeting?

- American-made carpets have not contained formaldehyde for decades?

- Formaldehyde will remain in cabinetry for years due to lack of fresh air?

- Diesel exhaust carbon is a major player in allergies?

- While humans might sneeze as a reaction to an allergen, dogs will scratch?

- The debris from oleander is poisonous, especially when it is dry and the tiny particles become airborne?

- Fragrances can act together with allergies to give an enhanced effect on the body and the mind and weather can enhance both of those effects?

- Indoor air pollution crosses all socioeconomic boundaries?

- Cancer causing agents are in our air and in our food?

- There is no such thing as deadly toxic black mold?

- There are probably more lawsuits in states with 200 mold spores per cubic meter of air compared with states that have 20,000 spores?

- That not buying various products will probably add more quality years to our lives and enhance our children's learning process?

- Breathing certain chemicals will cause children to act out?

- Television may be an asthma trigger?

- Paint odors are significantly more important than carpeting in a new home?

- Shopping for a home should include numerous environmental factors?

Contents

Section 1

Allergy Basics
pages 1–2

Section 2

Asthma
pages 21–22

Section 3

A Hazardous World
page 37

Section 4

We're Covered with Chemicals
pages 75–76

Section 5

Pesticides and Other Hazards
pages 105–106

Section 6

Indoor Air Quality
pages 139–140

Section 7

Pets and Critters
page 203

Section 8

Machines and Devices in the Home
pages 231–232

Section 9

Home Maintenance
pages 267–268

Section 10

Selling and Buying Your Home
pages 291–292

Section 11

Schools
pages 303–305

Section 12

Mold
page 325

Section 13

Safe Household Cleaning
pages 365–370

Section 14

Other Valuable Information
page 387

Preface

My interest in indoor air quality began in the late 1970s when I turned my attention from cancer research and university teaching to conducting IAQ tests for mold in the homes of allergic patients who lived in a farming community in Northern California.

When I began my company (Aero Allergen Research), in Tucson, Arizona in 1979, I began conducting a variety of tests indoors, and tracking the amount of pollen and mold indoors and outdoors that originated from numerous sites around the city. I had been hired to conduct the nation's first pollen and mold monitoring program for the purpose of pollen and mold control.

Sometime during those early years I sold one of our newspapers on the idea of carrying a column on the popular topic of the effects of weather on health and was actually hired by a television station to add the same information to their weather forecast.

This evolved into writing a weekly newspaper column on indoor air quality issues. The column continued for fifteen years. At one point I was appointed by the governor to serve on the air pollution hearing board, which dealt with larger issues such as the burning of used tires and others wastes.

My company grew and I decided to collect the vast amount of information I had accumulated over the years regarding IAQ and to put it into a crude volume that matured into this text. In doing so, the realization came to me that there is no spokesperson on a national level to represent the consumer on the hazards of today's indoor living. While I do not purport to be such a representative, it is my goal to ensure that as many people as possible read this book and practice what it preaches.

My records indicate that I have visited and monitored and inspected something like six thousand businesses and homes, from federal buildings, courthouses, jails, and drug vaults to trailers and million dollar homes. I have learned never to have any preconceived notions regarding what I might find and let the evidence or lack thereof speak for itself.

Yet there are common threads that connect them all—particles and gases, good health and bad health.

It was time for me to put events into motion and, with what can only be described as a labor of love, I completed this family resource guide for your referral and usage.

Introduction

Welcome to a new world of fewer sick days, fewer doctor visits, and better all-around health for you, your children, and your pets. In addition to feeling better, you'll benefit from a reduction in household costs as you eliminate cleaning supplies, the purchase of expensive equipment and personal care items that you don't need.

I have spent nearly forty years in the field of indoor air quality and give to you this book, which represents a tasting of recent and past reports of scientific data intermixed with my many experiences.

According to the American Lung Association, contamination from household products does not pose a serious health threat if it is both mild and brief. However, contamination often occurs over a long period of time and comes from a variety of sources. Effects can be serious, even fatal.[1]

A recent news report by Reuters described the findings of a new study published in the prestigious *New England Journal of Medicine*.[2] The investigators who conducted the study found that cleaner air over the past two decades has added nearly three years to the average American lifespan since 1980, five months of which they attribute to the reduction in fine particulate matter in the outdoor air.

While this is good news, it is at odds with the finding that asthma has increased by 58 percent over the past ten years, and that there has also been a strong increase in the incidence of cancer. Virtually all of this may have been caused by an increase in indoor air pollution, which is not associated with particles, but with a variety of chemicals, instead. One can only guess how much our life expectancy would increase if we reduced the fragranced products that we use in our daily lives.

Longer life is one reason why this book is important to everyone. It covers virtually every aspect of the parade of particle types we breathe and their sources of origin. It discusses the irritating gases that we are told will help us and which have just the opposite effect.

New information is always coming forth. From Europe comes a report that finds that even short-term exposure to diesel exhaust is associated with adverse effects in asthmatic airways, even in the presence of inhaled corticosteroid therapy. These particles appear in virtually all indoor samples collected from nearly every type of facility, even where air purifiers are present.[3]

This book applies to everyone. Where controversy exists, I discuss that controversy. And wherever you live, you will find valuable information in this volume.

Our vitality and that of our children is at stake. Think of yourself trying to function, trying to maintain a positive attitude on a smoggy day, or in a freshly painted room, or in a home that is strongly scented with formaldehyde. Picture yourself living in a house provided by our own government to victims of the Katrina disaster. The sad truth is that many, if not most of us, already exist under similar conditions. It might not be formaldehyde that is killing us, but a host of agents far more insidious and deadly.

This book is based on a collection of newspaper columns that have appeared over the past several years and enjoyed a readership of a half-million people weekly. I wrote the columns for the layperson, based upon my years of experience as the owner of an indoor air quality company, Aero-Allergen Research. The columns include facts gleaned from a myriad of publications in scientific journals and websites that belong to official organizations.

A number of chapters do not deal directly with airborne hazards, but are informative none the less. I would be remiss as a microbiologist if I did not include for the reader a general summary of microorganisms; or, as an air quality expert, if I did not write about how weather affects our health; or, about the significance of synergism on which I published my doctoral dissertation and scientific papers, and write about how it applies to our daily health.

Personal experience supplies a great deal of the information in this book. This includes years of inspecting and monitoring thousands of homes and businesses, and my own scientific research, much of which has been published in peer reviewed medical literature.

We have all witnessed a great number of technological changes in the last few decades. In many ways, the changes have not been in our best interest, and in many ways they have. This is certainly true in the field of respiratory health, which pertains to every person who breathes, not just to those with allergy and asthma. This book tells us what we can do to fix the problems at little or no cost.

Doctors and scientists tend to place blame on tight buildings, which resulted from the energy crisis of the seventies. Perhaps 90 percent of sick building problems are due to a lack of fresh air that would serve to dilute the contaminants. But it's more than that. There are no regulations regarding the sales of countless products to the home (or apartment) occupant. It's a seller's market in that few strong voices speak out on the side of simplicity. Some of those voices are listed in this volume.

Our ability to breathe safely affects our thought processes and our behavior. There is ample evidence to define this problem, and we can all understand it. What is in the blood goes to the brain. Why do children and adults undergo radical mood swings? Why are we depressed when we shouldn't be? Maybe it's due to the weather of the day, or an impending storm front, or maybe it is something more insidious. Hence, there is a section on weather and health, and an introduction of findings by Dr. Doris Rapp about schools and our children's behavior.

Greener Cleaner Indoor Air presents the basics of allergy and asthma, the chemicals we encounter in our daily environment, and their safe and inexpensive substitutes. It presents fundamental information about the home, apartment, or office, whether the structure is bought, sold, or rented. Do you want to know the latest information about ozone machines or any type of air cleaning device? Read on.

There exists a certain redundancy in this book. This is unavoidable, because the material it contains is interlaced and is important enough to repeat. Also, the reader may wish to review a general topic without reading about specific material in detail.

I use the term "toxic" in this volume, and I use it scientifically. It is not a generic term to refer to something vague. It refers to gases that harm the respiratory tract and neurological tissues, and cause a wide variety of effects that we are yet beginning to understand.

Small challenges can up to one large challenge. Allergens, added to fragrances, added to chemical odors, added to diesel exhaust, added to pesticides, can cause problems that may be hourly or may last years. Each of these additions saps our energy, our vitality, and our sexual desire. Together they work in synergy, where one plus one equals ten or one hundred.

To better illustrate this concept, let's rate our exposure to a given allergen or irritant on a scale of one to ten. Then, let's rank the amount of time we spend in contact with that element from one to ten and multiply this with the first number. An incidental exposure to a perfume at a low dose may yield a multiplier of one or two, while a heavy exposure over a longer period of time can give us a multiplier of fifty or one hundred. We can see how vastly different our exposure level can be, and we can expect a concomitant effect on our well-being.

The reference section provides an array of websites in keeping with today's world of information dissemination. I have also included a number of older classical scientific reports.

So much is available online that it is difficult to list all websites that are available to the casual reader who is interested in further researching the information presented here. Therefore, in many cases, I leave readers with general information that they can use to begin their own online research.

It is important to note that an incredible amount of the information readily on line is misleading and, quite frankly, stupidly wrong. Therefore, I suggest caution when researching any material presented on the Internet unless the source is credible. Sometimes it's hard to tell the charlatans from the honest presenter.

Given adequate research, valid authoritative materials are readily available for the reader to substantiate the statements presented herein.

The reader is cautioned about making inferences. For example, if one were to ask the question: If you were told that a certain level of pesticides had been identified in a given fabric, would you buy a garment made of that fabric? Or; if a certain mold was shown to produce toxins, would you be concerned about the presence of that mold in your home? Or: If an air purifier salesperson told you all the benefits of purchasing their product, would you do so without knowing the disadvantages?

In the first case, because we do know what pesticides were present in a particular garment, there is no way to measure the level that is absorbed into the body and the clinical effects of that exposure.

In the second case, we don't know if that particular strain of mold produces toxin and even if it did, its influence upon our health would be minimal at worst.

In the third instance, and except for the most extreme conditions and to this date, we don't have any clinical information regarding the effects of removing various particles or volatile organic compounds (VOCs) from the home or office air relating to clinical changes. In other words, is the patient better as a result of using this device?

In summary, there are too many overriding environmental factors in each our daily environments that affect us to enable us to obtain any meaningful information. All we can do is guess.

To follow all the recommendations in this book is to invite paranoia. Still, we should be aware of germs present on doorknobs, supermarket basket handles, refrigerator handles, and microwave doors.

My purpose here is to serve as a guide and as a general reference manual. There are countless topics that can be added to our subject list, such as extensive material relating to chemical sensitivity or electrical currents. Hopefully, the reference section will provide enough guidelines for interested readers to pursue their particular interests.

I have directed this information toward the mainstream public.

A note relating to opening of windows to permit fresh air to enter the home. This is not an absolute. This practice is counterproductive if pesticide spraying is occurring outside the residence, if a high number of pollen producing trees are near the home and it is pollen season, if agricultural areas are nearby which generate a high concentration of mold spores, if a weedy lot is present across the street and the wind is blowing in your direction. It is for each person to evaluate their particular circumstance regarding the weather of the day and the season when making a decision to exchange the inside air for the outside air. It is no different than making that decision based on freezing weather, stormy conditions or excessive heat. It only requires a little knowledge of the local environment.

Finally, the term *cubic meter of air* is used throughout this book. The term of cubic meter is standard notation in the world of science. A cubic meter is approximately twenty three percent or one-quarter greater than a *cubic yard.*

Additional Author's Note

We present an endless stream of requests for an endless supply of equipment.

We place orders for modern technology in the mistaken belief that it will provide a better education for our children.

We hold debates, PTA meetings, rallies, lobbies, sit-ins, strikes, political mayhem, and all manner of violent and non-violent protests to obtain funding in the misguided notion that allocations will create brilliance.

We demand that we allocate more money toward equipment for all levels of public and private education so that learning can improve and researchers can make more discoveries — as if equipment ever had the ability to make discoveries.

We support incompetent teachers because we accept incompetence.

We believe that money will create intelligence and inventiveness — even ideas.

None of these is true.

What we really need is just a few bold and marvelous researchers who have great honor and some nobility — a handful of thinkers with the makings of Aristotle, Kepler, Curie, Semmelweis, Pasteur, Koch, Tesla, Edison, and countless others who envisioned their goals and developed the means to reach them.

They took what existed and inserted their own ideas to fight the fight and forever change the world.

Let's lay some groundwork first. Then we'll see the truth: real thinkers can't be bought, but they can be created.

Endnotes

1. American Lung Association. 1998. Household Products—Indoor Air Pollution Fact Sheet. New York.

2. Pope A., M. Ezzati, and D. Dockery.2009. Fine-Particulate Air Pollution and Life Expectancy in the United States. *New England Journal of Medicine*. Vol. 360(4):376-386

3. Nordenhall, J. et al. 2001. Diesel exhaust enhances airway responsiveness in asthmatic subjects. *Eur Respir J.* 17:909-915

Section 1

Allergy Basics

Before we begin this section, let's look at some basic statistics:

Allergic diseases affect as many as 40 to 50 million Americans.[1]

Allergic rhinitis or hay fever affects between 10 percent and 30 percent of all adults and as many as 40 percent of children.[2]

More than ten billion dollars are spent each year on prescription medications to treat the disease.[3]

A nationwide survey found that more than half of all U.S. citizens test positive to one or more allergens and that 50 percent of homes had at least six detectable allergens present.[4]

In addition to allergic rhinitis, there are other types of allergy which include drug, food, skin, insect sting and latex. In addition, 55 percent of patients with sinusitis also had a history of allergic rhinitis with 18 million cases reported.[5]

Immunotherapy helps reduce hay fever symptoms in about 85 percent of people with allergic rhinitis.[1]

For our purposes, we will concentrate on aeroallergens or inhaled allergens, although I will present some basic information on a couple of other types of allergies as the book proceeds.

For most persons, exposure to allergens such as pollen, mold, cockroaches, cats, dogs, horses, and a witch's brew of others are of little or no consequence. For those tens of millions who are predisposed to allergy, however, initial exposure to allergens cause the production of allergic antibodies (immunoglobulin E, or IgE), and further allergen exposure may trigger an allergic reaction.

For those allergic persons who move to another city, it could take two to three years before their immune systems are "conditioned" to respond to the new environment. Hence, it is common for people to say that they never had allergies until they moved to a particular city, whether it is in a city or in the countryside.

Environmentally, numerous factors affect our reaction to our environment: the vegetation and traffic around the residence in which we decide to reside, our state of health at the time, our age, our relative location to traffic, the weather of the area, our change of diet, the age of the home, the lifestyles of the occupants who previously resided in the residence into which we are moving, our own lifestyles, and so forth. This is always true, whether we move or remain where we are.

Let's examine a few basics of allergy and see if we can apply these to our lifestyles and our health and make a little sense out of this mess.

Chapter 1
Allergy Q and A

Q. What is an *allergen*?

A. An allergen is a substance that causes the production of a certain class of antibodies that can lead to an allergic reaction. There are a lot of things we know today about what it takes to make an allergen that we didn't know a few years ago. For example, every protein has the ability to become an allergen.

Q. What is an *antigen*?

A. Antigens are chemical structures that can change a chemical substance, such as a protein, into an allergen. Thanks to the antigen, this allergen can elicit an allergic reaction. One way to remember it is that an allergen generates allergies and an antigen generates antibodies. Occasionally the terms will be used interchangeably (e.g., the chapter on cats).

Q. What does *sensitization* to allergens mean?

A. To become *sensitized* means that the immune response becomes primed to an allergen; that is, it becomes exposed for the first time. It is the first step in an allergic attack. Though sensitization often occurs during infancy, when the immune system is not fully developed, one can become sensitized at any time.

Some chemicals, such as formaldehyde may not be harmful over and above being irritants. However, they can act as a priming agent and sensitize the body to react to allergens.

Q. Suppose we are exposed to several allergens, such as *pollen, mold, cat allergen,* and *latex.* Are we more sensitive to allergens in general now that we have been exposed to more than one?

A. Yes. The greater the number of negative factors, the more sensitive we become. Negative factors include more frequent exposure to antigens, longer exposure to antigens, fatigue, heredity, and weakened immune response.

The immune response can be weakened by a number of factors, such as illness, depression, stress, poor nutrition, and exposure to *pesticides, steroids,* and *chemotherapy.*

The type of allergen is important. For example, many powerful allergens from certain pollen grains are released very quickly in the body; other weaker allergens are released more slowly. Those that are released more quickly can cause a rapid response by the immune system.

Q. What is a *cross-reaction*?

A. A cross-reaction occurs when antigens from different substances have a chemical structure that is similar. They share common antigens. For example, if you are allergic to birch pollen you can also react to latex *banana,* and *avocado.*[6,7] If you are sensitized to proteins found in certain pollen types, this could be a major reason for the development of food allergies associated with vegetables.

Q. How does air pollution affect the allergic response?

A. *Ozone* and *sulfur dioxide* are two pollutants associated with automobile exhaust. Latex is a pollutant associated with rubber tires (and thousands of household products as well). The first two enhance your sensitivity to allergens in general. Antigens in latex are also found in many foods and pollen types.

Chapter 2
Is It an Allergy or a Cold?

Although the symptoms are quite similar, allergies and the common cold are very different. Allergies are caused by an abnormal reaction against a normally harmless substance. The body reacts by releasing chemicals that bring about allergic symptoms.

There are six major types of allergies: foods such as strawberries, nuts or shellfish, skin (contact dermatitis), seasonal allergy (pollen and mold), allergy to pharmaceuticals (medications such as penicillin), allergic responses to pet dander (skin cells and shed proteins from oil-producing glands and saliva),and allergic reactions to insect body parts, stings, bites, and feces. All types have their own methods of triggering the body's immune system. General symptoms include sneezing, difficulty breathing, itchy or watery eyes, congestion, continual coughing, and dizziness. Severe allergies may cause vomiting or rashes.

In general, we can say that most allergies are seasonal; for example, they occur during pollen season in the spring or in the fall. If symptoms occur throughout the year, there is a good chance you are reacting to something in your home or work environment, such as a cat.

If you suffer from allergies, keeping a diary of the foods you eat and the substances you react to is always helpful. However, diagnosis may be tricky. Proper skin or blood testing helps doctors to prescribe proper medication. Many treatments are available for allergies over the counter or by prescription. Allergy shots, antihistamines, decongestants, sprays, and drops have been developed to minimize the effects of allergy symptoms. Allergies are preventable. The general rule for sufferers is avoidance.

The common cold, on the other hand, is brought on by an immune response that is triggered by a viral infection, usually entering through the nose or mouth. Most likely it enters those areas through direct means. For example, someone has a cold and touches the handle of the refrigerator, a doorknob, or a shopping cart. The next person comes along and opens the fridge or touches the same pushcart handle, then touches their nose or mouth. Children are prime suspects in this regard. A common drinking glass will produce the same result. Hand-to-mouth transference of viral particles is currently thought by many to be a more important source of infection than contact by sneeze droplets. (Please refer to the chapter on the spread of viruses and bacteria.)

Cold symptoms include scratchy throat, runny nose, sneezing, mucus drainage, watery eyes, and high fever. The risk of susceptibility increases during cold weather and when people congregate. For example, the start of a school semester will witness an increase in cold (and flu) symptoms. Also, people spend more time indoors during the winter, which means that chances of human contact are higher.

Susceptibility to a cold is high if the body is fatigued, distressed, or suffering from allergies due to a lowered immune system response. There is no cure for the cold, but there are many ways to prevent infection. *Hand-washing* is the most important, along with keeping hands away from the nose and mouth. Thinking about others in the family helps to prevent spread of the disease. Obviously, if it does spread, it is not an allergy, which is not communicable. Using common sense and maintaining clean habits, along with aerobic exercise and drinking plenty of fluids, are the best preventative measures. The best thing to do is relax and let your body fight the infection.

Chapter 3
Allergy Mysteries

Did you ever wonder how you could have a respiratory response to allergens even though you swore you were taking every precaution? Allergies are not so mysterious when we understand them better.

Cat allergen. More homes have cat allergen in their air than have cats.[8] It attaches to shoes and clothing from an area where there is a cat and travels to an area where there is none. You may have given up your cat, but it takes months, even years, for the antigen to disappear from soft furnishings and mattresses. Bird antigen is also long-lived.

I conjecture that there may be a link between library books, DVD rentals, and the transmission of cat, insect, and other allergen types. This is especially true if the book has been in an environment where cat, *house-dust mite,* and *cockroach* antigens are present. Books are intimate objects that we handle and take to bed with us. Maybe it's not just the old dust on books that makes us sneeze.

Latex. You got rid of your powdered latex gloves, but still have itchy, watering eyes. And now you have rashes as well. If you live near a busy intersection, you could be breathing in the particles that are shed from tires or particles of asphalt, both of which use latex as a major component. People who are sensitive to latex are frequently reactive to bananas, avocados, *kiwis,* and *chestnuts.* Thus, the allergic response takes the form of rashes.[6]

Sneezing upon waking. It's not pollen because the doctor told you to sleep with the windows closed, but you may have come in contact with an allergen before going to bed. It is not until four o'clock in the morning that natural biorhythms and resistance become low enough for bodily reactions to occur.

House-dust mites. Your skin tests show you are allergic to house-dust mites. You lower the indoor humidity to less than 45 percent to prevent their reproduction, which requires higher humidity, but you are reactive just the same. In this case, the dust mites became dormant to wait it out. But their feces are still present, and these are the particles that trigger the reaction.

Food allergy. You know you are allergic to wheat, so you don't eat it. You are still sneezing and have a sinus headache in the house. It's time to do some serious dusting and make the kids eat at the table. Allergenic food particles may be present in the dust we breathe. In some cases food antigens are in the smell of cooked food and in food particles that have fallen to the floor, to be ground underfoot and mixed with dust.

Sneezing upon walking outside. Do you sneeze when you go outdoors? Bright sunlight triggers photoreceptors in the eye, which activates nerves in the nose. It may not be allergies at all.

Chapter 4

Pollen

All flowering plants and grasses produce pollen. Some trees produce more than others and some kinds are more allergenic than others.

Pollen is the male contribution to plant reproduction. It is produced by male flowers and carried by various means to female flowers, which then become fertilized. The end result is a fruit, seed, nut, vegetable, or any number of edible and non edible products.

Pollen grains are microscopic and basically spherical. Most of them measure between twenty and seventy-five microns, about the size of many larger mold spores, and they can travel on the wind for miles. In general, 90 to 99 percent of them fall on their parent plant or within just a few feet of it. Wind can disperse a huge quantity of these grains within seconds or minutes once the gusts begin.

Pollen is allergenic because of the chemical structure of its coating, and because it releases growth enzymes upon striking a moist surface. The body of the allergic person does not recognize these new enzymes and reacts against them with an allergenic response. We call this hay fever. Hay fever is not a fever and is not caused by hay, although there was a connection at one time. Today, the medical profession refers to this condition as allergic rhinitis.

We know that both heredity and frequency of exposure to pollen can play a role in a person's reactivity. However, what makes some pollen grains more allergenic than others is not completely understood. For example, a person can develop an allergic reaction to ten ragweed pollen grains, but it might take a hundred birch grains or a thousand pine pollen grains to elicit a reaction.

Primary pollen allergens include ragweed and ragweed-related plants, grasses, birch, beech, cedar, ash, sycamore, and maple, among many others.

Colored flowers are less likely to release airborne pollen than are those that are not as showy. The colors attract insects, which carry the pollen directly to other flowers.

Generally, it is the wind-borne pollen that is allergenic, and the flowers that give rise to it must produce an incredible quantity in order to reach the female flowers on other plants.

Thus, it is primarily the wind-blown pollen that causes problems for us. That is why fields of wildflowers, for the most part, can be considered to be non allergenic. For one thing, they are just not that allergenic. For another, they are not readily airborne. That said, an overwhelming amount of pollen from any source can and will cause a sensitive person to react, and it may not just be the pollen, but also any plant and insect parts, mold, and other substances present during the pollen release.

Interestingly, I have found through personal observation that there is a 90 percent correlation between increases in airborne *Alternaria* mold and increases in the airborne release of many species of plant pollen twenty-four to forty-eight hours later. The spores are not only more numerous, but are darkened in their microscopic appearance. These correlations include ragweed, juniper, cedar, and other flowering plants. This finding may provide a predictive element to our knowledge of pollen forecasting.

Higher concentrations of pollen (and indoor mold) can be found in the air nearest the source. Because it is present on leaves and the ground near the plant, pollen can be picked up by breezes. Only a tiny percentage of pollen gets into the air, however. The remainder lies on the ground near the plant that produces it. The pollen can enter the house via air currents. However, it usually gets in when people track it indoors on shoes, or when pets carry it on their paws and fur, especially when they roll in the dirt. People also carry it indoors on clothing after yard work. That is why you should leave shoes at the door and doff outdoor clothing outdoors.

An indoor pollen problem can occur during the spring or fall months if there are several pollen producing trees in close proximity to your residence. Cypress, juniper, ash, birch, olive, maple, and sycamore are examples of trees that either produce copious amounts of airborne pollen, or produce lesser amounts of more allergenic pollen. In most parts of the country, ragweed plants produce billions of grains per plant of highly allergenic pollen.

A lesser number of pollen grains are produced by oak, the nut-producing trees, maple, mulberry, poplar, aspen, mesquite, paloverde (southwest), and numerous other species. These may be highly allergenic, but only present in small quantities in the air. Again, any tree pollen may be allergenic to a sensitive person, especially if the trees are located close by.

Depending on where you live, pollen is a big problem between the months of July and October, when allergenic weeds and grasses are abundant. It may appear as early as February in the desert southwest. These pollen grains enter the home by tracking as well. Solution: remove your shoes at the door.

Thunderstorm asthma is a term that has been used for many years and has been described in more detail recently. There are a number of studies that have linked either pollen or mold with the disease.[6-11] Thunderstorm asthma refers to the fact that asthma worsens during and shortly after a thunderstorm, as measured by hospital admissions. In one case, raindrops strike a pollen grain such as rye grass. Grass has starch granules within each of the tiny grains that are subsequently released. While the pollen grain itself is not small enough to reach the deeper lung spaces to trigger an attack, the starch granules are (i.e., less than five microns). Each grain can contain as many as 700 starch particles, all of which are antigenic. The pollen can be in the air or it can still be in the *anthers* in the grass for this to occur. In addition, the granules can also attach to diesel exhaust particles, which now serve as a vehicle to carry the antigen into the lungs. An increase in allergic symptoms also occurs during this period.

In the case of fungal spores, rainfall triggers the release of numerous spores almost immediately. The smaller ones are inhaled. At least one study has found that turbulent winds could increase the release of fungal spores or draw up sediment fungal spores and resuspend them in the air, making them available for inhalation.[11]

Chapter 5

Hay Fever

The National Center for Health Statistics (NCHS) reports that twenty-five million adults and children had hay fever in the year of 2008.[12] Billions of dollars a year are spent on hay fever medications.

Allergic rhinitis, **or** *hay fever,* is different from asthma. It is not life threatening, but can be an expensive disease when one takes into account the cost of medications, time, and doctor visits, and impairment of performance efficiency at home, school, or work. Its symptoms are nasal itching and congestion, sneezing, and red, itching eyes with tearing. Quite often the patient has the feeling of general fatigue and just doesn't feel well. Frequently, these symptoms can be traced back to lack of sleep.

Employees with this illness sometimes take a sick day; if they do not, there is a chance that their work won't be up to their usual standards. Loss of sleep may contribute. It is ironic, but inexpensive medical care is part of the problem. For fifty years people have been able to obtain *antihistamines* without a prescription. Of the working men and women who have hay fever, half use over-the-counter antihistamines. These medications cause drowsiness and make us mentally and physically slow. The side effects may be worse than the disease.

In today's world, new medications such as non-drowsy or non-sedating antihistamines are readily available over the counter. They last longer than the medications of old and are quickly gaining in popularity.

We can see why it is very important for doctors, parents,

teachers, and school nurses to be aware of the fact that hay fever can impair a child's ability to learn. They should also be aware that it is possible for a child's behavior to be affected by a particular medication, but not by another.

Chapter 6

Other Common Allergens

Foods. The foods most likely to elicit an allergic response are shellfish (shrimp, crab, lobster, snails, clams, and oysters), peanuts and tree nuts, tomatoes, eggs, milk, soy, and wheat, although potentially, any food substance can be a candidate, depending on the individual's sensitivity. Reactions to food can typically include, itching, rashes, swelling of the lips and throat, diarrhea, vomiting, and severe respiratory distress. It can be life threatening.[13,14] A person may react to a vegetable such as a tomato when it is eaten raw, but not react to it when it is cooked. In addition, even a trace amount of the food substance may trigger a reaction.

Feathers. The most common source of feathers in the home is a *pillow.* Allergic individuals should use pillows made of *Acrilan* or *Dacron*, which will last a lifetime with proper care. For best results, enclose them in a dustproof cover to prevent house dust from settling into the stuffing. You can obtain these covers from drugstores, from department stores, or by special orders online.

Cottonseed. Most inhalant allergy traced to cotton comes from particles of cottonseed. These are commonly found in the stuffing of *pillows, sofa cushions, mattresses, bed pads, blankets, and upholstered furniture.* If you cannot eliminate these items, cover them with dustproof covers.

Outside the home, cottonseed is found in some cattle and poultry feeds. Additionally, most miniature golf courses are covered with ground cottonseed mixed with other substances.

While cotton may still retain the residue of one or more pesticides, cotton fabrics are commonly treated with formaldehyde for permanent-press and fireproofing purposes.

Pyrethrum. This is the dried flower of the pyrethrum plant, which is a member of the *chrysanthemum* family. Chrysanthemums and pyrethrum are closely related to *ragweed*. Thus, ragweed-sensitive patients may also experience symptoms upon exposure.

Pyrethrum is a common ingredient in insect powders and sprays for the house, garden, and pets. It is also very popular for use in mothproofing carpets, draperies, and upholstery, as well as preventing the growth of insects in these materials. It is advisable that the pyrethrum-sensitive patient not go into rooms or closets that have been recently treated, and that they do not wear clothes that have been recently mothproofed. This substance is also found in ointments.

Pyrethrum sensitivity can be seasonal and *hypo sensitization* by an allergist may help.

Sulfa compounds. Many insecticides that are used out-of-doors contain sulfa compounds.

Sulfating agents. These are added to foods to retain color and freshness (Please see the chapter on Asthma Triggers.)

Some allergists question the relationship of these pesticides to sulfa-related allergy.

Orris root. One can obtain orrisroot by powdering the root of this plant, which is related to the iris. It is often used in cosmetics, scented soaps, toothpowders, bath salts, perfumes, shaving creams, and lotions. Its scent is what makes it attractive.

At one time this substance was thought to be allergenic. Today, it is of little interest to allergists and they do not perform skin tests for sensitivity to it.

Endnotes

1. National Institute of Allergy and Infectious Diseases *Airborne Allergens: Something in the Air.* NIH Publication No. 03-7045. 2003.

2. The Diagnosis and Management of Rhinitis: An Updated Practice Parameter. Joint Task Force on Practice Parameters. *J Allergy Clin* Immunol 2008; 122:S1-S84.

3. Soni, A. *Allergic Rhinitis: Trends in Use and Expenditures, 2000 to 2005.*Statistical Brief #204, Agency for Healthcare Research and Quality. 2008.

4. Arbes, S.J. et al. Prevalences of Positive Skin Test Responses to 10 Common Allergens in the U.S.Population: Results From the Third National Health and Nutrition Examination Survey. *J Allergy Clin Immunol.* 2005; 116:377-383.

5. Hamilos, D.L. Chronic Sinusitis. 2000. *J Allergy Clin Immunol.* 106:213-27.

6. Alenius. H., K. Turjanmaa and T. Palosuo. 1995. Cross-Reacting Allergens in Natural Rubber Latex and Avocado. *J Allergy Clin Immunol.* Aug; 96(2)167-173.

7. Makinen-Kilijunen, S. 1994. "Banana Allergy in Patients with Immediate-type Hypersensitivity to Natural Rubber Latex: Characterization of cross-reacting antibodies and Allergens". *J Allergy Clin Immunol.* Jun;93(6):990-6.

8. American Lung Association. 2009. Allergy Statistics and Facts. http://www.lungusa.org.

9. Suphioglu C. 1998. Thunderstorm Asthma due to Grass Pollen. *Int Arch Allergy Immunol.* May 119(2):37.

10. Dales, R.E., MD, et al. 2003. The Role of Fungal Spores in Thunderstorm Asthma. *Chest* March 24.

11. Pache G.E. and Ayres J.G. 1985. Asthma Outbreak During a Thunderstorm. *Lancet* 2:199-204.

12. National Center for Health Statistics. 2008. Allergies/Hay Fever. Summary Health Statistics for U.S. Children: National Health

Interview Survey, Appendix III, Table V. http://www.cdc.gov/nchs/fastats/allergies.htm.

13. American Academy of Allergy www.aaa.org.

14. American Academy of Allergy, Asthma, and Immunology www.aaaai.org

Section 2

Asthma

This series on asthma has been adapted from a lecture presented by Michael A. Kaliner, MD, as presented in a booklet by the U.S. Department of Health and Human Services, National Institutes of Health and Infectious Diseases. I would also like to thank Dr. Jacob Pinnas (retired) of the Allergy and Asthma Center of Arizona and former head of the Pollen and Mold Committee of the AAAAI, and Dr. Gerald Goldstein (retired), Diplomate of the American Board of Allergy & Clinical Immunology, for their contributions.

According to the United States Department of Health and Human Services, bronchial asthma is among the most common chronic diseases.

Let's look at some asthma statistics:

Approximately 34 million Americans have been diagnosed with asthma by a health professional during their lifetime.[1-3]

Workplace conditions, such as exposure to fumes, gases or dust, are responsible for 11 percent of asthma cases worldwide.[4]

About 70 percent of asthmatics also have allergies.[4]

The prevalence of asthma increased 75 percent from 1980-1994.[5]

Children 5-17 years of age missed nearly 13 million school days due to asthma in 2003.[5]

In a survey of U.S. homes, approximately one-quarter had levels of dust mite allergens present in a bed at a level high enough to trigger asthma symptoms.[6]

Approximately 40 percent of children in the United States who have asthmatic parents will develop the disease.[1,6]

The prevalence of asthma in adult females was 23 percent greater than the rate in males in 2006.[7]

Asthma often recurs when former sufferers reach their thirties, and many others still have abnormal airway disease.[8]

The disease can be managed through education, avoidance of triggers, and medication.

This section will present information about the disease in terms of its basics, some medications, and a little about its management.

To me, the knowledge of the spectrum of asthma triggers is quintessential for the asthma patient. The knowledge of what triggers onset of the disease is foremost to avoidance of its causes, early management, and follow-up treatment.

Chapter 1

What Is Asthma?

People often think of asthma as a relatively benign disease, but about five thousand Americans die from asthma each year. Asthmatics of all ages are at risk, and while children might outgrow the disease, it can return when they enter their thirties.[8,9]

Asthmatics have trouble breathing due to secretion of excess mucous, contraction of the smooth muscles that line the airway, inflammation and swelling in the airway, and muscle spasms. Triggers include the usual irritants, such as airborne allergens (aeroallergens) and dust, chemical smells, tobacco smoke, and even automobile and diesel exhaust. Vehicular exhaust gases and their attendant carbon particles frequently enter indoor workspaces, houses, hospitals, and schools in particular, where idling diesel school buses are the predominant culprit.

Asthma is not a problem with breathing *in*, but with breathing *out*. During normal inhalation, air moves smoothly from the mouth through the trachea, bronchi, and bronchioles into the alveoli. If you're an asthmatic, you can do the same: you lower the diaphragm and swing your ribs out, making the lungs bigger.

However, breathing out is not active, but passive. Ordinarily, all you do is stop breathing in, and you automatically breathe out. But if you're an asthmatic, you can't do this. The minute you relax your ribs, the obstructed airways block the airflow, and air can't get out. Used air space is trapped in your lungs. You end up breathing at the top of each lung rather than using the entire lung.

If you don't have asthma and want to get a sense of how it feels, try this: Breathe in. Now don't let the air out. Hold that deep breath and breathe in and out using only the tops of your lungs. That's what an asthmatic experiences. Now get out of breath through exercise and try the same thing.

When an asthmatic's airway is full, it contains not only excessive, very sticky mucous, but also a lot of other debris. This includes white blood cells. The airway becomes irritable and sore. When asthmatics cough, inhale cigarette smoke, or inhale other irritating *fumes* or *vapors*, they may begin to wheeze—a whistling sound that occurs because the irritable airways are now constricted.

Chapter 2
Asthma and the Office

Avoiding asthma-causing substances and situations in the home is one thing. Doing the same thing at work is a different challenge altogether. Though stress at work is certainly a leading trigger for an asthma attack, the physical environment also plays a large role.

It is common for many people to occupy a room meant for only a few. This can happen when a small-to-medium-size office is turned into a conference room, lunch room, teaching room, or lounge. Several things can occur as a result. First, in an air-conditioned building, there is a buildup of carbon dioxide and a decrease in the amount of available oxygen when rooms are used for other than their intended purpose. Engineers try to balance air flow to each room and if an office meant for two or three persons is converted into a conference room, not enough fresh air enters through the air supply registers for the number of people who are working.

This scenario is compounded when many *copiers, computers,* and other electronic machines are packed into a particular area. When the airflow in these rooms is not designed for such a dense concentration of humans or machines, as is often the case, the end is a higher occurrence of asthma, along with *headaches, drowsiness, irritability,* and other symptoms.

Because there is not enough recycled and filtered air for a dense concentration of workers, the particles that are tracked in from outside also build up. Add to this various microbes from cold and *flu* viruses that come from the workers themselves.

In a closed space, such as an *airplane* or an *office* environment, diseases are more easily transmitted through the air.

It is important for management to take proper dilution of indoor air into account and permit specialists to adjust and balance the airflow to account for the increase in the number of people. The issue occurs not only in offices, but also in hospitals and classrooms.

Businesses in many parts of the country rely on roof-mounted evaporative coolers for their indoor cooling. When these devices are in place, numerous problems can arise. These include asthmagenic (asthma-causing) odors derived from mold and bacterial growth.

Other triggers involve an obvious exposure, such as a chemical spill, or an environment that is too hot, too dry, or too cold for comfort. This is because the smooth muscles of the airways are sensitized in the asthmatic patient and become easily irritated.

Problems with asthma in the workplace commonly appear after the weekend or after a vacation, when a return to the office represents a change in the environment. Symptoms can appear after less than an hour in the workplace, within two to eight hours after starting work, and even at night.

Chapter 3

Types of Asthma Medications

A note of caution: If you are on prescription medication, you must take only that which is prescribed for you. Do not take something a friend or neighbor gave you to try out.

Cromolyn. This drug helps prevent allergics. It is used in an inhaled form for asthma and in a nasal spray for allergic rhinitis. It stops the *mast cell* from secreting the chemicals that cause allergies. Cromolyn does not work for everybody, and it is expensive. But for anyone with allergic asthma, this drug is worth a try and may prevent exercise-induced asthma.

Bronchodilators. These relax the smooth muscles that line the airways and open the airways. There are three classes of bronchodilators: anticholinergics, methylxanthines, and beta adrenergic agonists.

> » *Anticholinergics* relax the large muscles around the bronchi (large airways). These muscles tighten making the airway narrower. The medications blocking the concentration of *acetylcholine*, a neurotransmitter, which triggers the muscles to contract. These are medium-strength drugs with a shorter duration of action than adrenergic agonists. They may be used for the treatment of patients who produce excess mucous. They take 20-30 minutes to have a good effect, but the symptoms can be alleviated for 24 hours.

> » *Methylxanthines* have become popular in the last twenty years. This class of drug is the most common type

used in the United States for the treatment of asthma. The best known methylxanthine is *theophylline*. Theophylline acts by stopping some of the enzymatic actions in smooth muscle cells, thereby relaxing them. This is a potent form of therapy that can have very serious side effects if its concentration in the blood rises too high due to the effects of other drugs, fever, flu shots, or diseases.

» *Beta adrenergic agonists:* Beta receptors are found in various cell types throughout the body including the lungs. Stimulation of these receptors in the body by adrenaline can have a variety of effects. Beta adrenergic blockers inhibit the normal reactions of adrenalin and their use can result in a reduction in blood pressure in those asthma patients who are hypertensive. The best part is that several of these drugs are more specific for the lungs and usually do not affect the rest of the body, although they may cause tremors or cardiac stimulation in some patients. Beta adrenergic agonists work within minutes and can prevent exercise-induced asthma.

Corticosteroids. These are probably the most effective drugs for the treatment of asthma, especially when it is out of control with worsening symptoms. They work by reducing swelling, reducing mucous secretion, reducing numbers of mast cells and secretions, and even by stopping the production of the IgE allergic antibody. However, research suggests that they may decrease attention span in children and produce insomnia in some adults. Recently, there has been some concern that certain other drugs or fever can interfere with elimination of corticosteroids from the body, allowing its concentration in the blood to rise and become unsafe.

Inhaled steroids have been engineered over the past several years to work in the nose and lungs, with little action in the rest of the body. They are usually considered to be safe and effective.

Immunotherapy (allergy shots). This is useful when asthma has clear-cut allergic causes that are not readily controlled with medication. When immunotherapy works, it reduces not only the need for drug therapy, but also helps treat the disease itself.

Chapter 4

Asthma Triggers

The number one *asthma trigger* is allergy. About 90 percent of children under ten who have asthma also have allergies. If you are younger than thirty, there is a 70 percent chance that you are allergic.[9]

Allergists tell us that about 75 to 80 percent of the air a healthy person inhales is exhaled within one second of maximum exertion—that is, breathing out as hard as possible. By three seconds, the lungs have essentially emptied. Asthmatics can't breathe in as much because all their air is trapped in the back of their lungs. Even at six and seven seconds they are still blowing out air. This is one way your doctor can determine if you have the disease.

An allergic reaction works in the following manner: Every tissue in the body has *mast cells*. These cells are most heavily concentrated in the mucous membranes (the skin that lines the nose and the airways). When mast cells are sensitized by having *IgE* (allergy-related) antibodies on their surface and they encounter that antigen or foreign substance, this triggers the release of histamine and other agents from inside the mast cells, which, in turn, causes the allergic reaction.

At first, you don't exhibit an allergic reaction until you have been exposed to the antigen (pollen, mold, dust) for a certain period of time. So if you just acquired a cat, just wait!

For example, ragweed produces about a billion pollen grains per plant per year. After two or three seasons of breathing in an allergen like ragweed pollen, (and after IgE has attached to the mast cells), the mast cells will release histamine and other chemicals. Asthmatic and allergic reactions now occur. This reaction will happen to an asthmatic who is allergic to certain foods. That's one reason why people with allergies commonly complain that their allergies become active again after they have moved to a new location, but only after a couple of years. They blame it on the location. They are only partly right. Their immune system becomes sensitized to the new antigens (allergens) and by the second or third season of exposure, they are now responsive to those antigens.

Allergies are often hereditary. According to the American Lung Association, if you are a parent with allergies, the probability is that one in three or four of your children will have allergies. If both parents are allergic, all offspring can expect to be allergic.[9]

When is allergy likely to be a contributing factor to asthma?

It is likely when a blood relative has allergies.

It is likely when the asthma begins at a young age.

It is likely when the asthma symptoms occur or worsen seasonally, such as the fall or spring.

It is likely when other allergic symptoms also occur, such as rhinitis (runny nose), hay fever, or *eczema*.

It is likely if tests show that blood and sputum contains an increased number of *eosinophils*.

Infections can also cause asthma. *Bronchiolitis* is a viral respiratory infection that occurs in children younger than two. A child may get a bad cold and then develop respiratory distress. About half of these children, if they have an allergic parent, will go on to develop asthma; thus, the viral infection is the primary cause of asthma exacerbation. Generally, this asthma is fairly mild and greatly improves before the child is ten years old.

Some asthmatics only have asthma symptoms in relationship to a cold and sinus infection. You will recognize sinusitis because you feel mucous dripping down the back of your throat, and your throat may feel sore. Frequently, you will have pain in the sites where the sinuses are located and develop headaches. You may run a fever. Sinusitis commonly causes asthma to worsen.

Nighttime asthma can occur when stomach acid backs into the esophagus and irritates its lining. Thus, *acid reflux* may be a trigger. This event sets up a reflex action in the chest, triggering an asthma attack. Overeating or eating the wrong foods may play a partial role.

Cigarette smoke and other chemical irritants can trigger asthma, as can intense emotions and psychological stressors. Triggers also include rapid temperature changes, onset of stormy conditions, and cold weather.

Recognize that airborne pollen levels are usually highest before noon, when flowers open in response to sunlight, as well as when winds begin to increase. Indoor air that is filtered from a central system, and even evaporative cooling during pollen season, may help you escape the highest concentrations of the allergens.

Industrial and occupational exposure can lead to asthma. Inhaled substances (particulates) can act as allergens, or as irritants (chemicals) that do not result in IgE production. The most common cause of occupation-related asthma is the inhalation of substances like *toluene, benzene, acetone, xylene,* or *formaldehyde.* Anyone who inhales chemical vapors can develop bronchial irritation and become sensitive to the chemical. It is estimated that as many as 15 percent of asthmatics develop asthma in response to industrial or occupational exposure.

Very common triggers of asthma are nonsteroidal anti-inflammatory drugs such as *aspirin*. Aspirin is a very potent drug and about 5 to 10 percent of asthmatics have asthma that is triggered by aspirin or other aspirin-like compounds. These include *indomethacin, phenylbutazone* and *ibuprofen*.

One group of chemical additives that triggers asthma attacks in susceptible people is sulfites, commonly found in wines. *Sulfiting agents* are commonly added to foods, such as salad ingredients, to keep them from turning color and to act as antimicrobials. They have been used since the mid-1600s and, until recent years, have been regarded as safe. Asthmatics serve as an exception. Today the Food and Drug Administration requires labeling of sulfite-containing foods and prohibits salad-bar restaurants from adding sulfites to their fresh foods. However, processed foods at salad bars may still contain sulfites; the same is true of meats and fish. Approximately 5 to 10 percent of asthma sufferers have a sensitivity to these agents. Those who are on steroid treatment are especially sensitive, as are women.[10,11]

Beta blockers (beta adrenergic antagonists) have been recognized as triggers for asthma since their first day of introduction. These chemicals are used for treating *migraine* headache, *glaucoma*, rapid heart rate, high *blood pressure, tremors*, and other conditions. You may need to switch to an alternate drug if you have asthma. Talk to your doctor. Beta blockers can make your asthma worse, according to the U.S. Department of Human and Health Services. This is why it is important not to change dosages without your doctor's approval. Even taking medication the same time of the day is important so that the proper blood level can be maintained.

Exercise is a potent stimulator of asthma. When people exercise, they *hyperventilate* by taking rapid, shallow breaths. Just as evaporating water cools the skin, hyperventilation cools the airways. A reflex reaction to this cooling of the airways causes an asthmatic reaction. *Running* is the worst exercise for asthmatics due to the rate of expiration of water vapor, and *swimming* is the best because they inhale moist air, slowing down the cooling of the airways.

Wearing a surgical mask can enable a person to re-breathe humidified air. More than 8 percent of the athletes who represented the United States in the 1988 Olympic Games had exercise-induced asthma. Proper medication helped them maintain a close check on their disease. Consequently, they made it through years of rigorous training to the highest level of competition.

Idiopathic (unidentified) triggers of asthma occur in about 25 percent of asthmatic individuals over thirty. Here, the exact triggers are unknown. This type of asthma occurs most often in older individuals who have some bronchitis, a lot of excess mucous secretion, and perhaps sinus infections.

In summary: Asthma is commonly allergic in nature. A trigger can be of varying strength. It can be particle, an odor, or a food. A person will react to a cat allergen before they will react to a dog allergen because the former is more potent.

Dehydration is often a cause of an asthma attack.

The proper medication can be used preventively and can be used to ease an attack when it does occur.

Education and a doctor's care are important tools for management of the disease.

Endnotes

1. Sommer E. et al. 1998. "Global plan launched to cut childhood asthma deaths by 50 percent. *National Institutes of Health.* December.

2. National Institutes of Health. 1990. Review of *"What you Need to Know about Asthma"*, by Michael Kaliner, M.D., Allergic Diseases. Department of Health and Human Services. **www.nih.gov.**

3. American Lung Association. 2009. *Allergy Statistics and Facts.* **www.lungusa.org.**

4. World Health Organization 2007 Global Surveillance, *Prevention and Control of Chronic Respiratory Diseases: A Comprehensive Approach.* **www.who.int/en/.**

5. Akinbami, L. *Asthma Prevalence, Health Care Use and Mortality: United States 2003-05,* CDC National Center for Health Statistics, 2006.

6. Arbes, S.J., et al. House dust mite allergen in U.S. beds: Results from the first national survey of lead and allergens in housing. *J Allergy Clin Immunol.* 2003:111:408-414.

7. American Lung Association. Nov. 2007. Epidemiology and Statistics Unit, Research and Program Services. *Trends in Asthma, Morbidity and Mortality.*

8. Levinthal, B.G. 1986. National Jewish Center for Immunology and Respiratory Medicine. *Your Child and Asthma.* **www.nationaljewish.org.**

9. American Lung Association. 2009. *Allergy Statistics and Facts.* www.lungusa.org.

10. Lester, M.R. 1995. Sulfite sensitivity in human health. *J Am Coll Nutr.* Jun:14(3):229-32.

11. Gunnison, A.F. and D.W. Jacobsen. 1987. Sulfite hypersensitivity: A critical review. *CRC Crit Rev Toxicol.* 17(3):185-214.

The websites for the National Institutes of Health, (**www.nih.gov**), American Lung Association **www.lung.usa.org**),World Health Organization (**www.who.int/en/**), American Academy of Allergy Asthma and Immunology (**www.aaaai**), (as well as their links), can be immensely helpful in providing virtually all the information the inquisitive mind would want or need to know regarding the relevant topics.

Section 3

A Hazardous World

The purpose of this section is to present some basics regarding our present state of health and where we can go in the future and will add to our longevity. What we have done to ourselves, on purpose, by accident, or what we have been introduced to without our knowledge is another issue.

From particles to gases, we live in a virtual sea of respiratory irritants. We purchase many of them with the best intentions, and others enter the house on air currents or on the bottoms of our shoes. Because of this, the EPA recognizes that the environment within our homes, workplaces, and schools may be ten times as hazardous to our health as the outdoors. Fortunately, in most cases, there are a lot of easy fixes and the fixes don't involve buying things, but involve *not* buying things.

The average reader might be astounded as to the number of hazardous chemicals to which we are exposed on a daily basis. Once we see this, the vast majority of the chemicals can be eliminated very easily through alternate purchases, or no purchases at all.

Chapter 1

Household Dust

The vast majority of indoor allergies are caused by house dust. People with house dust allergy usually feel worse when indoors, during the night, and they suffer year-round. They generally feel better when out-of-doors. Just what is this stuff that causes perennial allergic rhinitis, bronchial asthma, and respiratory allergy?

I have found that house dust is a complex mixture composed of fragments and feces from organisms such as *moths, cockroaches, ants, silverfish, spiders, mites, plant hairs*, and *flower parts* that are tracked indoors; pollens and spores; fibers of material made from cellulose such as *cotton, linen, jute*, wood, and *kapok*; manmade fibers such as fiberglass, *nylon, plastic*, Dacron, rubber, and a dozen others; animal and human hair and skin cells; cigarette smoke, *fireplace soot* and *diesel exhaust* carbon; *lead, insecticides*, and *aerosols* from personal care products; and cat and dog antigens. House dust may also include food particles (such as allergenic wheat products) and tracked-in outdoor dirt that contains various minerals and becomes worn to a powder.

According to the American Lung Association, contamination from household products, if limited to low levels for short periods of time, does not pose a serious health threat. However, contamination can occur over a long period of time from a variety of sources. Effects can be serious, even fatal.[1] For example, in recent years, a number of harmful products have found their way into the home, and therefore into the house dust. These in-

clude cleaning furniture products, spot removers, oven cleaners, rug and upholstery cleaners, air fresheners, moth repel-
lants, hobby materials, glues, and many others, most of which
are volatile organic chemicals (VOCs).

If you are curious, you can sift through your carpet cleaner
bag to see larger examples of the particles you're breathing.
These settle on the heater to get burned in the winter. Multiply
them by the number of times you must empty the bag each
year to get a rough idea of the amount of dust that accumulates
in the average household.

The biggest problem children in this house-dust family are
mite feces, cat antigen, cockroach parts, animal *dander*, and
mold spores. The amount depends on your living conditions
and location.

Humans shed about one gram of skin cells per day. Mites
survive on this dander, as well as on the shed dander of animals.

The worst areas of the home for house dust are the soft
furnishings, deep pile carpeting (especially hard to vacuum),
unmopped wood or tile floors from which dust is readily airborne, upholstered furniture, *drapes, stuffed animals, blankets,*
and *bedspreads* of all types. Usually, the older the furniture, the
more allergy it causes. This is because there is a deeper layer of
dust in older furnishings, and a large reservoir of dust mites.
The dust on the TV screen is held there by *electrostatic* means,
and other than affecting the clarity of the picture, it is not considered to be an airborne dust threat.

That there is lead in household dust is a major discovery. The
amount can vary from low to high within and among homes.
Infants and children are more likely to get lead poisoning than
adults due to the continued development of their nervous system. Infants crawl on rugs and carpets with dust (and lead),

then put their fingers and hands in their mouths, transferring the lead. Further investigations will likely reveal that adults also have problems caused by this element. One possibility is that substantial lead exposure during childhood can increase blood pressure during young adulthood.[2]

Low-level exposure to lead causes a decrease in IQ. Lead exposure is also associated with speech and language problems, increased aggressiveness and acting out, reduced attention, and lower scores in reading, spelling, and math. It is quite likely that there is no safe level of lead exposure.

Some decades ago, people became concerned about dust in the home and decided that it was better to keep it out because it aggravated allergies and triggered asthma. As technology improved, we started looking for different substances in dust and found them.

The next breakthrough in the field was the ability to detect many of these substances in the human body, determine how much of each was there, run tests on people, conduct surveys, and determine what these particles and gases were actually doing to us. We started to make some discoveries and got a few surprises.

Now we are starting to look at combination effects, where exposure to two pesticides yields a hundredfold or a thousand fold or greater increase in human-tissue-effects.

The rates of *cancer* and various respiratory diseases have been increasing in the United States. In past years, much more money was directed toward outdoor air pollution, although we spend 90 percent of our time indoors. In recent years this trend has reversed to more correctly address the real experience. Our exposure to toxic substances indoors is five to ten times greater than our exposure outdoors. In some cases it is a hundred times higher. This includes exposure to pesticides, lead, heavy metals, and cancer-causing volatile compounds. Most of the problem is associated with two types of hazards: those that start in the indoor air and end up in house dust, and those that start in outdoor dirt and end up in house dust.

Don Aslett maintains that dusting should precede vacuuming. This is because a clean, well-maintained vacuum cleaner will not leak dust into the air, and that cleaning a house involves a lot more than dusting; it involves dislodging dirt particles, which can then be removed by vacuuming.[3]

In theory this sounds fine. However, with the use of electronic equipment, I have found as much as a tenfold increase in airborne dust during vacuuming by the vacuum cleaners he has tested. This was due to the turbulence created at floor level. The faster the movement, the more turbulence is created.

In conclusion, it would appear that it doesn't matter which you do first, as long as you do it slowly and carefully. Only then do you stand a good chance of reducing clinical symptoms.

Chapter 2

Soft Furnishings

Soft furnishings retain a high level of dust, which includes the highly allergenic cat antigen. Take a sofa pillow outside, stand upwind, and beat it to see what I mean. According to data I have obtained, every time someone sits on a soft furnishing, it releases a cloud of dust into your breathing space and may produce ten to one hundred times the level of dust that was initially present in the air.

If you are in the market for furniture, look for solid unwoven or tight-weave fabrics. These may be cotton or synthetic and will retain very little dust. You might want to ask about the amount of formaldehyde in the wood frame of the chair or sofa, and in the fabric itself, though the salesperson might not know. Formaldehyde recently made national news as a serious eye and respiratory irritant; it was present in high concentration in mobile homes that the federal government provided for Hurricane Katrina victims.

Another option is to shop for an appropriate cover for that old sofa or chair. This is more economical than buying a new one.

With the use of a particle-counting meter that measures six different sizes of dust particles, I have found that vacuuming can raise the level of airborne dust from ten to a thousand-fold if the vacuum cleaner is leaky or the person cleaning uses it improperly. Sometimes it is better not to vacuum than to vacuum. Certainly, carpeting can add visual warmth and serves as important insulation in many homes. Importantly, it offers protection for infants in homes, schools, and day care centers who may fall onto the floor.

Household dust settles near the walls because of its tendency to swirl outward as we walk. Concentrate your damp dusting (or vacuuming) at the floors' edges.

A bed can be covered with a nice-looking tight-weave blanket to catch the dust; this can be carefully folded back at night. If your bedspreads aren't too large, you can put them in the dryer on air or tumble cycle to remove dust. Otherwise, you may have taken them outside, weather permitting.

Unfortunately, the presence of snow and ice does not cut down on indoor dust, as we continue to track it in with the slush on our shoes and boots. Tracking is the primary means through which dust enters the home, so leaving shoes at the door is an important method for the reduction of household dust.

Venetian blinds should be vertical, not horizontal, to minimize the amount of dust that settles on them. Curtains, drapes, and lampshades should be smooth and solid, not porous or rough.

If you minimize the number of soft furnishings or cover them with an easy-to-clean material, you minimize dust and allergens. Simplicity is the key to success in significantly reducing the amount of dust in your home and making housecleaning easier. Sometimes just a little reorganization is all that is necessary.

Chapter 3

Sleeping with a Window Open

Weather permitting, many allergic people sleep with a window open at night for fresh air. They believe that because most trees and many weeds release pollen during the day, there will be few respiratory hazards when they breathe the cooler and fresher nighttime air.

What really happens is that much of the pollen remains airborne due to the presence of air currents. In addition, the cooler and denser air mass in the morning hours slides down mountain slopes or contours of the ground to settle into low-lying areas of the community. Anybody who has driven a motorcycle down into a dip in the road will recall cool air masses.

These settled air masses can be a thousand feet in height or much less, but they can bring down with them aeroallergens that have built up in the atmosphere during the day. Outdoor dust can do the same thing, as the particles combine with pollen, mold, vehicular exhaust carbon, and a variety of particulate pollutants, causing them to settle out at a high concentration.

Additionally, during pollen season, a clinically significant amount of pollen is usually present at all hours of the day or night, though more of it is present during peak hours.

To summarize, whether you open a window for fresh air at night depends on the season and location. Living near a busy intersection is different than living in a spread-out residential community. The presence of a lot of trees in the neighborhood will reduce the spread of vehicular pollutants, but you must also take into account the fact that these trees may produce allergenic pollen during the spring months.

Chapter 4

The Fireplace: Problems and Solutions

In 1998, 18,300 residential fires in the United States originated in chimneys, fireplaces, and solid fuel appliances, according to the United States Consumer Products Safety Commission. These fires resulted in 160 personal injuries, forty deaths, and $158 million in property damage.[4]

Changing pollution standards around the country are causing a phase-out of wood-burning fireplaces. If you still use one, then you need to know how to avoid breathing the toxic wood gases and how to prevent your soft furnishings from absorbing them.

Several factors can lead to fireplace smoke entering the home: If the air is very cold outside and your fire is slow to start, then there will be insufficient heat to break through the plug of cold air in your chimney. A larger quantity of smoke will enter your home. The remedy for this is to hold a wad of lighted paper into the chimney throat to warm the air before you light the fire.

Many people go to bed with the fireplace still burning. If the fire dies and the house cools off enough in the early morning hours, this will cause a suction of air down the fireplace, and any remaining smoke will enter the house. Tightly closing the flue at night will alleviate this problem as long as the fireplace is cold.

In newer homes, if the forced-air furnace starts while the

fire is going, it will create negative pressure inside, pulling air into the furnace to be circulated throughout the home. Kitchen and bathroom fans can have the same effect if they are on.

Downdraft can also occur for the following reasons: The chimney is too short. Trees, hills, or nearby buildings deflect the wind downward. The chimney is older and does not meet code. The fire is too large, and the chimney has not had a chance to warm up. Or, finally, there is no open window on the windward side of the house.

Check with your local wood-burning fireplace outlet for the latest in technology, or check online to help to eliminate drafting problems.

Burning wood always gives off carcinogenic creosote, especially when it burns incompletely.[5] It is also flammable when it accumulates in the chimneys of older homes, and it is more likely to accumulate if too much wood burns too fast and combustion is incomplete. If you burn plastic, it will stick to the inside of the fireplace. The burning of foil, painted wood, or garbage in the fireplace can also result in the production of poisonous fumes.

Hardwoods, such as ash, beech, birch, maple, and oak provide a longer-lasting fire with a shorter flame. Avoid burning wood that has been treated with chemical preservatives (or binders), as they will be released back into the home along with the smoke. These chemicals are also harmful to the metal and structure of the fireplace.

Ideally, you should cut the wood you use in the spring so that it is dry by winter. This way the moisture content will be less than 20 percent, and the wood will burn more completely. Heat energy will not be lost vaporizing the water.

If you have a gas line stub to your fireplace, then you can use special gas logs. Gas is a much more efficient fuel in terms of heat given off per dollar spent. Using it helps you avoid all the problems of wood burning—greater fire danger, allergenic and asthmagenic smoke entering the home, the purchase or cutting of the wood, and the cleaning of the unit. Unvented gas appliances are similar to other fire-producing appliances, however, in that that they become less efficient when there is poor ventilation, as in an airtight newer home. Less efficiency means that the gas logs will produce poisonous carbon monoxide gas.

The pellet stove is an exciting new heating technology. The stove burns sawdust waste from sawmills, compressed into pellets about the size of rabbit food. A gravity feed drops the pellets into a closed combustion chamber. A fan provides air circulation, and the stove vents burned gases outside. Very high temperatures are reached with this method of burning because the pellets are dry, and combustion is virtually complete. It is considered to be the cleanest wood-burning technology to date.

Pellet stoves can be freestanding or inserted into fireplaces. Mobile home units are available. The production of toxic gases in the home is not an issue with pellet-burning devices because the stoves burn them completely and vent the gases which will not enter the home.

An approved fire extinguisher should always be handy near an open flame, or when you use high heat.

The Fireplace: Hazards

Wood smoke can reside in soft furnishings for months. The smoke has a lot of different components. Let's look at a few of them.

PM-10. These are very small particles less than ten microns in size (particle mass less than ten *micrometers* or microns). Smaller than pollen grains, they can deposit more deeply in the lung, where some of them remain indefinitely to cause damage. Rapid declines in lung function can occur upon exposures to PM-10s. The smaller particles can cause the most lung damage.[6] The gases mentioned below can attach to the particles to compound the problem.

Studies published in the mid-1990s revealed that a particle size of 2.5 microns could cause serious health problems. The number of particles this size has decreased in the outdoor air over the past two decades, contributing to longer life spans.[6]

Carbon monoxide (CO). CO combines with hemoglobin, the oxygen-carrying substance in the blood, replacing the oxygen. This suggests that people with angina or atherosclerosis should not use wood-burning fireplaces, as they may produce CO, and this will affect the area of the heart that requires oxygen-rich blood. Clinical symptoms include lethargy, drowsiness, dizziness, nausea, fainting, and headaches. These symptoms are similar to flu and food poisoning. An overdose of carbon monoxide can lead to death.

Aldehydes (including formaldehyde and acrolein). Both of these are present in wood smoke. According to published scientific data and information provided by the EPA, exposure to formaldehyde above 0.4 parts per million is associated with upper airway irritation, headaches, and disorders of the nervous system. Also, it is presumed to be a carcinogenic risk to humans. Acrolein is an even more active irritant of the eyes and respiratory tract.

Nitrogen oxides (NOx). NOx are known to cause a buildup of fluid in the lung at high concentrations. They are comprised of a mixture of *nitrogen* and oxygen and are released into the air through the exhaust of motor vehicles and the burning of coal, oil, or natural gas. Children from homes with gas cooking stoves (which emit NOx) have a greater frequency of respiratory illness than do children from homes with electric stoves.

Polycyclic aromatic hydrocarbons (PAH). Many of these compounds are carcinogenic in animals. They also include chemicals that result from the burning of scented trees such as juniper, cedar, pine, and eucalyptus.

All of the above chemicals are present in the air and furnishings of homes that burn fireplace wood. Obviously, the burning of *plastics, textiles, laminated wood,* and other materials can worsen problems.

Chapter 6

House Fires

Expect smoke from a fire to go anywhere that air goes. The soot and the odor are toxic to different degrees in different people, or the same person at different times. This is true of any respiratory irritant. Good restoration of the home after a fire means removal of soot and odors.

The first step in odor removal is to get rid of its source. An ozone machine is used to produce the gas at a very high concentration (beyond human tolerance) to oxidize and ionize particulates that are in the air. The ozone molecules attach to the particles and gas molecules so the smell is no longer present. This permits the cleanup crew to spend time in the dwelling without having to wear respirators. After that, they may use a deodorizer to mask any remaining odor. (Please refer to the chapter on Ozone.)

Most people are shocked at how much and how long their lives are disrupted after a fire occurs. Even if the fire is small, expect to do some or all of the following: cleaning carpets, *window coverings*, bedding, furnishings, and clothing; repainting *walls* and *ceilings*; restoring oil *paintings* (including frames and backings); repairing *windows*; cleaning and replacing electronics and computer systems; discarding foods (other than canned goods); and replacing medications and *cosmetics*. You may have to remove furnishings and clean them inch by inch with a cotton swab.

Failure to clean the furnace, air conditioner, cooler, and/or ductwork could result in the release of soot back into the home when the air-handling system is turned on.

In short, virtually everything will have to be cleaned or replaced.

Ideally, you should prepare a list of household items before anything happens, along with photographs, just as a precaution. Maintain this file outside of the home or in a fireproof box. Though the entire process is lengthy and tedious, it will come in handy if a fire does occur: fire restoration specialists can refer to your list and help you determine which items can be cleaned and which items should be replaced.

Unless the restoration process is done correctly, the smell and the soot will remain, emitting low to moderate concentrations of toxic gases for weeks, months, or years. Residents, pets, and visitors to the household will experience exposure during these emissions, both through inhalation and absorption through the skin. The smell and soot may also decrease the resale value of the house.

It is important to note that fire from synthetic materials is likelier to contain more dangerous gases than fire from natural materials. Synthetics include most carpets, chairs, sofas, beds, wallpaper, and wall paneling. It is especially dangerous when plastics and materials from hydrocarbons are burned. These include products with *Styrofoam*, formaldehyde, *nylon*, and polyvinylchloride (PVC). The gases they release include *phosgene*, *cyanide (found in Styrofoam)*, and *hydrochloric acid*. Fire department handbooks speak of hundreds or thousands of chemicals that are created when synthetic materials burn.

The presence of smoke from a fire can not only impair vision, but also lead to loss of consciousness and irritation of the entire respiratory tract. It can cause physical weakness, loss of coordination, heart issues due to angina, faulty judgment, blurred vision, and panic. Survivors of a fire may also experience a variety of lung-related problems after the event.

In addition to gases that result from the smoke, particles in liquid form are suspended in the air and on surfaces. Known as *aerosols,* they can be viewed under a microscope at two hundred to five hundred times magnification, and they can be enumerated. Even if you've cleaned every surface after a fire, the liquid droplets can remain suspended in the air, numbering in the thousands to tens of thousands per cubic meter of air. They are liquid irritants and liquid carcinogens. Thus, every corner of the home must be air-flushed after "final cleanup" has been performed.

If a fire has occurred in your residence, it is important to ensure your health by consulting with businesses that specialize in fire cleanup. If you are experiencing symptoms as a result of the fire, consult with your doctor.

Much of the information in this chapter has been supplied by the current National Fire Protection Association/Fire Prevention Handbook, with the kind assistance of TM Building Damage Restoration, Tucson, Arizona.

Chapter 7

Candles: Soot and Aroma

Carbon soot comes from a variety of combustion sources. These include fireplaces, *water heaters, furnaces, pilot lights*, smoke from cigarettes, *cigars*, and *pipes*, cooking byproducts, *gas dryers*, automobile exhaust, and fires in general. Other carbon-related particles come from the burning of plastics, and from roof and street tarring.

An additional source of carbon soot—one people may not expect—is candles. In fact, a trend toward candle purchases has contributed to an increase in household soot. Candle technology, or the lack of it, is partly to blame for the problem. First, manufacturers tend to increase the amount of aroma in a candle. A common result is incomplete combustion and a rise in both soot and volatile organic compounds (VOCs). When amateur candle makers produce inferior-quality candles for the home, they can produce the same effects.

With a candle there is a tradeoff—brightness for soot. The brightness of a candle depends on two factors: the volatility of the wax, and the yellow-white part of the flame. This color of flame is relatively cooler than the hotter blue part of the flame. Soot is formed by incomplete combustion of the *candle wax* as it burns in the cooler yellow-white part of the flame.

The bigger the *wick* is, the bigger the flame will be, and the brighter the candle will burn. This means that it will release more soot. Wicks that curl as they burn remain short and hot, but not very bright. Carbon soot from candles will be present throughout the home, but mostly in the room in which they burn.

There is an interesting effect called "ghosting," in which the fine soot particles are attracted to some areas of the home and not to others. For example, while *sheetrock* (or *drywall*, or *gypsum board*) may darken, the nail heads that hold it to the studs do not. Areas behind pictures may remain clear of smoke, while shapes appear on the walls and ceiling. The association of soot particles with electromagnetic lines of force in the home may be the reason for the shapes.

Some homeowners report that they have removed carbon with simple soap and water. Others state that they had to completely repaint to restore the interior.

Partially opening a window should alleviate the problem of carbon soot buildup.

Many of those who recommend burning herbs for treatment of asthma also recommend the burning of candles or incense containing extracts of *cajeput, hyssop, cypress, myrrh, eucalyptus, lavender, frankincense, lime, juniper, spearmint, ragweed, and spruce.* For thousands of years, different types of therapy have revolved around using these plants. However, inhalation of these vapors or fumes is not healthy for persons with allergies and lung disorders, as they are not only allergenic but also asthmagenic.

Any scented candle can trigger an asthma attack. (Please refer to the section on fragrances.)

Chapter 8
What Is Radon?

Radon is a colorless, odorless, naturally occurring radioactive gas associated with *uranium* deposits. Uranium deposits occur widely in the Earth's crust and are found in the soil of all fifty states. Once in the soil, the gas can move to the air or migrate to the water below the Earth's surface. Because it is a gas, radon attaches to dust particles, which people can then inhale.

Uranium deposits are most common in *granite, shale,* and *limestone.* Uranium decays into radium, and then into radon, which quickly decays into a half dozen isotopes. Radioactivity is released at each conversion.

Radon can migrate via limestone cracks in the earth to locations distant from its source. When it enters the home, it does so through the following locations:

» cracks in floors and walls
» gaps in suspended floors
» openings around sump pumps and drains
» cavities in walls
» joints in construction materials
» gaps around utility penetrations such as pipes and wires
» crawl spaces that open directly into the building

It may also dissolve in well water.

On May 9, 2008, the EPA reported that radon is the leading cause of lung cancer among nonsmokers and, like cigarette smoking, long-term exposure increases the risk of lung cancer.[7] Unlike smoking, radon does not cause short-term health problems such as coughing, shortness of breath, headaches, or fever.

The EPA originally wanted 40 percent of all residences tested for radon gas by the year 2000. As of that date, only about 7 percent of homes had been tested. Since then the issue has become less important, however the EPA still recommends that you test your home because of hot spots in the country that are known and unknown.

Though levels of radon are low outdoors, they can be high indoors. This is because the gas tends to accumulate in basements where it enters, in most cases. Homes with no basements tend to have much lower radon concentrations, as do homes with evaporative cooling, which causes forced exiting of the home air.

A picocurie is a measure of radiation. Short-term tests for radon can be carried out over two days to provide the picocurie concentration in your home. The measure of four *picocuries* per liter is the federal standard for the maximum concentration that should be present. During these tests, the house is closed as much as possible. Though these short-term tests are not very accurate, they are popular because they provide a quick answer. More accurate testing should be performed over the course of three to twelve months. Two canisters should be used in all testing cases. In these long-term tests the home need not be closed, and the residents can enjoy normal living conditions. Testing over the long term frequently gives much lower readings.

Radon test kits are available from the National Safety Council; (call 1-800-SOS-RADON). Some home improvement and hardware stores also sell test kits.

At this time, the issue of radon's effects on health has not been resolved to the satisfaction of many investigators.

Chapter 9

Asbestos: How Hazardous Is It?

Some say that the main problem with asbestos is not with on-going hazards to its exposure, but the publicity about its hazardous potential.

Asbestos is an extremely small, naturally occurring fiber. Unlike fiberglass, it is not absorbed when it enters the lungs. Excessive exposure to asbestos usually takes years to develop into a disease state. Many workers who were involved in the manufacture of products containing asbestos developed asbestos-related lung disorders twenty to thirty years later and died. These disorders, known as asbestosis and mesothelioma, are cancer related. Mesothelioma is a disease of the mesothelium, the cell layer that lines the internal organs. There are numerous on-line sources that discuss these diseases in detail.

The EPA tells us that from the 1930s through the 1970s, asbestos was heavily mined and widely employed in homes, schools, and office buildings.[8] Products that contained asbestos included insulation for steam pipes, boilers, and furnace ducts; vinyl asbestos floor tiles and adhesives; patching and joint compounds, artificial ashes and embers sold for use in gas-fired fireplaces, various paper-related products as insulation around furnaces; door gaskets in stoves and furnaces; soundproofing (popcorn ceilings); joint compounds; roofing shingles and siding; fireproof gloves; stovetop pads; and automobile brake linings. Some houses built between 1930 and 1950 used asbestos as insulation. It was not used in acoustic ceilings (popcorn) since the early 1980s when existing stocks were used up.

According to virtually every source, however, no respiratory hazard exists as long as there is no effort made toward the substance's removal. This is the essence of the problem.

The amount of airborne asbestos resulting from its removal from a household is extremely minimal compared to the original worker-exposure levels. That said, you should still make contingency plans regarding asbestos removal if you are buying a period home and plan to remodel. Just keep in mind that doing so can be a lot more expensive than leaving things as they are.

Disposal of asbestos can include scraping, grinding, or sanding vinyl flooring and its mastic down to the slab, removal of popcorn ceilings, or unwrapping it from steam pipes and heating sources. Older asbestos will crumble when handled, so don't handle it. In those cases, call a professional asbestos removal company. If you are going to remodel and remove the popcorn ceiling, it is recommended that you spray ample water on small patches of the ceiling and scrape off the area with a blunt knife. These samples should be submitted for analysis. If no asbestos is found, you may continue your work. Otherwise, call in the professionals to complete the project.

Watch out for companies that tell you removal is the only way to go. Repainting a ceiling that has asbestos can be accomplished with a low pressure sprayer, but check around for alternate methods. Ask your experienced hardware dealer for ideas.

In addition, overlaying a vinyl flooring on top of another vinyl flooring is much more expedient, cheaper, and safer than removing and replacing the entire floor and having to deal with asbestos in the vinyl or in the mastic. Wrapping older piping with aluminum tape, aluminum foil, or even duct tape is another inexpensive method of containment.

Again, schools and houses with asbestos in structural materials are not at risk, as long as those materials are not disturbed. Removing it from schools that have no issue of airborne asbestos is a huge waste of money and may do more harm than good.

Chapter 10

Fiberglass

———

Simply put, fiberglass forms when liquid glass is extruded through tiny holes, then cooled.

Unlike asbestos, fiberglass is a synthetic product. It is derived from silicon and used in thousands of products ranging from surfboards to insulation in attics, air ducts and air-handling closets, air filters, and wall insulation.

Under the microscope, its form is quite distinct from that of other fibers. Natural fibers such as cotton and wool are broad and vary in width with frayed ends; synthetic fibers like nylon and rayon are uniform in width, with ends approaching ninety degrees. Fiberglass, however, reflects light, is spearlike and straight, and doesn't fold over or bend as the others do.

Occasionally, when it is the shape of loose cotton ball-like flocking and in high airborne concentration, the fibers will be inhaled; this can lead to coughing. Also, when the glass particles come in contact with skin, eyes, and nose, they can cause itching and irritation.

If fiberglass is present in an attic where recessed lighting is in place, pressure changes may permit it to enter the home proper. Also, air duct leakage will pull in the surrounding flocking, sending it into a room where it will become part of the dust.

Fiberglass loses its ability to insulate (its R value is decreased) when it gets wet or becomes exposed to high humidity. However, once it becomes dry again, it regains its R value.

It will not support the growth of mold unless the material

is old and dusty, or the paper backing on non-flocking-type insulation is wet for an extended period of time.

The *NIOSH* (National Institute for Occupational Safety and Health) *Guide to Chemical Hazards* handbook states that fiberglass health concerns may arise when the airborne level reaches three fibers per cubic centimeter. This is in relation to persons who work with the product and inhale it. That's equal to three million fibers per cubic meter of air. The average home may have only a tiny fraction of this number, that is, from none to perhaps one hundred *per cubic meter* of air, although exceptionally poor construction may lead to exceptionally high levels. The good news is that it takes a lot of fiberglass to cause problems. The problems I have observed are related to itching when the particles are emitted from the air handling system or loose flocking from the attic or crawlspace or behind drywall when exposed to air currents. Coughing due to the presence of fiberglass particles in the air is a rare occurrence in the domestic or office setting, in my experience.

Chapter 11
Electromagnetic Fields

The effect of electromagnetic fields (EMFs) on people has been under investigation since the late 1800s. There is a great volume of international literature on the topic that indicates slight trends rather than definitive results. The use of cell phones as a cause of brain tumors is still under investigation.

There are two classes of EMFs. The first class belongs to those waves that are part of the electromagnetic spectrum (similar to visible light) with longer wavelengths. These include radio and television signals, microwaves, and radar.

The second class includes magnetic waves that are generated in our environment when electrical appliances are used. As one might expect, as we move from area to area within our home, the strength of these waves will vary depending on our proximity to the appliances, the strength of the wave (field) the appliances generate, and other factors.

Sometimes within a tight home, the electromagnetic lines of force can be seen on walls, where carbon soot from candles may deposit.

One problem with studying the effects of EMFs is that there is no way to accurately measure tissue response after exposure, as we are not magnetic beings.

Another problem relates to statistics. Do we have enough cell phone users in our sample to determine whether they have a higher occurrence of brain cancer than nonusers? How do we know that people who live under power grids or high-voltage towers didn't work for power companies at one time and prefer to live there? Is the slight increase in the number of leukemia cases in electrical workers due to the electric fields in their workplace environment or the chemicals used in the manufacture of the products? These are the questions science must try to answer.

Complaints by people who claim sensitivity to EMF include redness and burning of the skin, fatigue, dizziness, nausea, heart palpitation, and digestive disturbances. Most research, however, indicates that individuals with electromagnetic hypersensitivity (EHS) cannot detect EMF exposure any more accurately than non-EHS individuals. Well-controlled studies indicated that symptoms were not correlated with EMF exposure.[9] According to one study, psychosomatic illness could not be ruled out.[8] Investigations in this area are ongoing in the field of EMF production by electronics and further research may find that their presence may have a real effect on the human.

The amount of electrical energy that is produced by small household appliances (measured in milligausses) drops off dramatically as distance from the appliance increases. Thus, the effect on a person may be ten to one hundredfold less than it is at the source, such as a radio, computer or toaster.

If EMFs lead to problems for the average person, it may be that they are acting as a stressor rather than causing a measurable disease. As such, it may be appropriate to add it to the long list of stressors in our environment, the sum of which probably contribute to our well-being, or lack thereof.

Our electronic age has surrounded the average person with electromagnetic fields of a wide variety of strengths, many of which occur indoors. Studies of the possible effects of ELF (extremely low frequency fields) on health are hampered by problems in measuring exposure and by the great degree of exposure in the community.[10] The jury is still out on the real effects of EMFs on pregnancy, health, sleep, attitudes, and behavior.

The Chemical Injury Information Network (CIIN) has available material on EMFs for the interested reader.

Chapter 12

Traveling by Car

To ensure that your car does not affect your health adversely, here are a few suggestions.

- Steam clean the engine periodically. The smell of hot grease and oil under the hood have a tendency to enter the vehicle.

- Check the caps on the *radiator, brake fluid,* and gas tank for tight sealing and replace them if necessary. Improperly sealed caps permit hot gases and volatile liquids to escape into the car's interior.

- Ensure that the air filter is clean. This will allow the entry of fresh air into the engine for more efficient gas combustion and better fuel economy.

- Keep track of your mileage. You can do this by writing down the number of miles registered on the odometer when the tank is filled, then noting the mileage the next time you fill up. Divide the total number of miles traveled by the number of gallons it took to fill the tank. (You do not have to use an entire tank's worth to check the mileage; half a tank will do. Just make sure to fill the tank each time.) If the mileage begins to decrease, then the car may need a tune-up.

- Inspect the entire exhaust system for leaks. This includes areas around the muffler, as exhaust fumes will enter the car from there.

- If you plan to carry solvents and cleaners in the vehicle, make sure that they are tightly sealed.

- During spring or early summer, driving with the windows down in an area of heavy tree density will permit high levels of pollen to enter the car. Keep the windows up and set the airflow to "recycle." When the AC is on, or when the vents are open and the windows closed, car passengers are only exposed to a small percent of the outdoor aeroallergen particle load. Exposure is much higher for both front and rear passengers when the windows are open.[11]

- If you are shopping for a new car, first see if you get along with the high concentration of odors emitted by plastics, adhesive, and fragrances.

- Follow at a safe distance behind vehicles that are "smokers."

- At the car wash, be wary of fragrance strips that are added to the rearview mirror, or fragrance sprays that might be added to the interior during the initial cleanup.

Chapter 13

Traveling by Commercial Airplane

Though hundreds of millions of people fly each year throughout the world, there is a curious lack of information regarding specific illnesses caused by air travel. One reason is that people become ill for various reasons after exiting the plane and don't report their illness to the airline. If they did, there would be little to nothing the airline could do about it unless there was a massive outbreak of some respiratory virus.

At the risk of going into too much detail, we will use the Boeing 737 as an example and discuss its cabin airflow parameters. [12]

Typical pollutants that must be confronted are the usual: dust, pollen, lint, smoke, bacteria, and viruses. The airlines are not deaf to the concerns of their passengers and attempt to stay current on methods to deal with air-quality issues. In this regard, they have installed cabin air filters and are introducing true HEPA (high efficiency particulate air) filters as an upgrade. The latter are capable of removing virtually all but the smallest particles (viruses) from the air and are designed to operate for six thousand flight hours.

The main problems people encounter within a commercial aircraft have to do with airflow and pressurization. During flight, the environmental control unit of the aircraft conditions the air for heating, cooling, and ventilation. Then a pressure-control system establishes the internal cabin pressure as a function of altitude. This pressure is maintained at an altitude equivalent of eight thousand feet. This is three-fourths of the available oxygen pressure at sea level, but is still fairly comfortable. (To maintain the cabin at sea level pressure would put unreasonable demands on airplane structure, fuel, and finances.) This pressure is maintained, even if the aircraft is at forty-one thousand feet. Hence, there is more difficulty in breathing for many who fly.

One might think that longer flights would saturate the air with water vapor from respiration, but the opposite is true. One of the biggest problems aircrews have on long-haul flights is dry air. During the process of taking in outside air that is very cold (and very dry), the air is also run through a device that takes removes any water vapor. This prevents ice from forming and showing up in the air ducts.

The resulting lack of moisture is especially problematic on longer flights, when the air outside consists of pockets of ozone that can enter the cabin, and the amount of available oxygen decreases as people move around more. Dry air has become such an issue that some pilot unions have actually negotiated to have humidifiers available in the cockpit.

A full cabin air exchange occurs every two to three hours. The airflow ducts are distributed evenly throughout the cabin, moving the air from front to rear. There is recirculation of air in an effort to save gas, but fresh air is added throughout the cabin and exhausted out the back of the jet.

In the past, air was filtered through a HEPA-like system that was small enough to filter out bacteria, but not small enough to filter out viruses. Newer filtration systems utilize true HEPA filters, which have a better filtration capability. The tradeoff is this: by minimizing the amount of fresh air that enters the cabin, the airlines save fuel, but bacteria, viruses, and particulates remain airborne for a longer period of time.

In a building containing two hundred employees, the ventilation system would have to provide four thousand cubic feet of fresh air per minute to prevent respiratory ailments and infections, headaches, drowsiness, and coughing, and to carry away respiratory irritants such as perfumes, other personal care products, and volatile organic compounds in general. That comes to twenty cubic feet per minute (CFM) per occupant recommended by ASHRAE. (In 1924, the rate was only four CFM.) The ventilation rate of the 737 is 1,900 CFM, or about thirteen CFM per passenger in a full plane that holds approximately 146 passengers.

In summary, numerous factors potentially affect passengers' health. These include confined atmosphere and a buildup of particulates and microbes, low humidity, reduced oxygen, and exposure to occasional outside pockets of ozone, which may become heightened in concentration inside the cabin for several minutes. All of these can affect fatigued or jet-lagged passengers.

With improvements in technology, commercial airplane manufacturers have taken strides toward improving the air quality of the cabin while endeavoring to keep fuel costs (and ticket prices) low.

Endnotes

1. American Lung Association. 1998. *Household Products-Indoor Air Pollution Fact Sheet*. New York.

2. Gerr,R., et al. 2002. Association between Bone Lead Concentration and Blood Pressure Among Young Adults. *Amer J Ind Med*. Aug:42(2):98-106.

3. Aslett, D. 1982. *Do I Dust or Vacuum First?* Writer's Digest Books, Cincinatti, Ohio.

4. Environmental Protection Agency. 2008. *Wood Burning Efficiency and Safety*. **www.epa.gov/woodstoves/efficiency.**

5. Fears, F.W. *Field and Stream Wilderness Cooking Handbook Globe* Pequot. Pg. 13.

6. Environmental Protection Agency 2008. *Particulate Matter (PM10)* **www.epa.gov/air/airtrends/aqtrnd95/pm10.**

7. National Safety Council. 2009. *Frequently Asked Questions about Radon*. http://www.epa.gov/radon/pubs/physic.

8. EPA. 2009. *Asbestos*. Feb. www.epa.gov/asbestos

9. World Health Organization. 2005. Fact Sheet #296. Our Toxic Times May 2006. *Electromagnetic Fields and Public Health*. Chemical Injury Information Network. Great Falls, Missouri. **www.ciin.org.**

10. Coleman, M. and V. Beral. 1988. A Review of Epidemiological Studies on the Health Effects of Living Near or Working with Electricity Generation and Transmission Equipment. *Int J Epidem* 17(1):1-13

11. Muilenberg, M.L. et al. 1991. Particle Penetration into the Automobile Interior. I. Influence of vehicle speed and Ventilation mode. J *Allergy Clin Immunol* 87(2):581-585.

12. Boeing.2009. *Commercial Airplanes: Air Quality*. www.boeing.com/commercial/cabinair.index

The Chemical Injury Information Network (**www.ciin.org**) is a support and advocacy organization dealing with multiple chemical sensitivity. They offer referrals to experts in the areas of electro-magnetic fields, less-toxic pesticide usage, and a wide variety of other areas. Their monthly newsletter is a helpful guide to keep the reader up to date on the latest in new discoveries and government approaches to environmental problems.

Section 4

We're Covered with Chemicals

In today's world, the average person is the target of a vast marketing system. As a result, we are covered literally from head to foot with untested or poorly tested fragrances, *chemicals*, *sprays, body lotions*, and *preservatives*. International reports have decried the promotion of products so pleasing to our sense of smell that the consumer cannot connect with the fact that they are used as pesticides first and perfumes and colognes second and that even our pesticides are fragranced. Read the labels and you'll see what I mean.

A listing of reported symptoms related to these chemicals is almost ludicrous. I invite you to make up an ailment—any ailment; there's probably a perfume or fragrance that can be linked with it. Even occasional contact or inhalation of these substances may cause a clinical reaction.

The information in this section is critically important for the health and longevity of adults, children, and pets. I will present only a small portion of information from the available literature.

As you will find, most of the scented products are meant to make our lives easier, more enjoyable, more relaxing, sexier, and more healthful. Just the opposite is true in the vast majority of cases. In this section we will examine some of the most common of these cases and wonder how we ever got into this mess. Most importantly, we can find out how to get out of it, saving our money and our health at the same time. Some excellent references will guide the reader to learn more about this subject which I consider an epidemic of global proportions.

Chapter 1
The Material Safety Data Sheet

There are complex federal requirements concerning material safety data sheets (MSDSs) for toxic chemicals. Employers must provide an MSDS to employees when a hazardous chemical is used in the workplace. Normally, businesses will provide an MSDS to customers upon request, but only upon request. Paint stores and pest control companies are two common businesses that maintain one or more MSDSs on their products.

The MSDS contains a lot of scientific and medical information about a product's chemicals in their purest form, as well as in their final diluted form.

Let's take a look at what MSDSs have to say about fragrances. Fragrances are frequently used to mask other smells, and are supposed to have a pleasant smell of their own. One common type of fragrance used in athletic clubs is billed as an odor neutralizer. Its purpose is obvious. The MSDS for this product states that it contains *methylene chloride, ethyl alcohol, methyl alcohol,* and *anisobutane* and *isopropane* blend. The MSDS tells us that this product is nonflammable, but that the container should not be exposed to temperatures above 130 degrees or it may explode. No problem so far.

If we read on, we find out that this product can decompose into hydrochloric acid (muriatic acid for swimming pools), carbon monoxide, chlorine, and phosgene. Phosgene gas is created when chlorine is mixed with carbon monoxide, and it has been a known respiratory irritant since the early part of the twentieth century. This product is a simple *asphyxiant* if vapors are trapped and inhaled, and overexposure to the "odor neutralizer" can lead to mild eye irritation, headaches, dizziness, nausea, possible unconsciousness, and even death. Much of this information is for workplace production of the chemical and its integration into the "odor neutralizer" packaging, but it is still available for the end user—the consumer—to evaluate.

A second MSDS describes the ingredients in a popular furniture polish, which contains petroleum distillates and mineral oil. The MSDS states that it should not be mixed with other chemicals. It is flammable. It is not expected to irritate the eyes, but may cause skin irritation. Prolonged exposure to high vapor concentrations of this product may cause headaches or dizziness. Affected persons "normally" experience complete recovery when removed from the exposure area. This product is not expected to be toxic by ingestion. However, if this material is swallowed and aspirated into the lungs, chemical *pneumonitis* may result. An affected person should be moved to an uncontaminated area and get medical attention, and the area of product usage should be fresh-air flushed.

The Internet is a good way to find a particular MSDS of concern. The interested reader may just want to type in the initials MSDS and then search for the one of concern.

Chapter 2
Perfumes and Fragrances

For thousands of years, countries like Persia, India, China, Egypt, Greece, and Italy (Rome) have used perfumes and other fragrances. Uses have included prayer, worship, air purification, eradication of evil spirits, induction of self awareness, cures for insomnia, reduction of allergy and asthma symptoms, and numerous other clinical and psychological applications.[1,2] However, the credit for the first use of inhalation therapy goes to Egypt.

In Asia, incense is used for small food establishments to keep out flies.

In 1986 the National Academy of Sciences (NAS) targeted fragrances as one of six categories of chemicals that should be given high priority for neurotoxicity testing.[3]

Perfumes are an international problem. In 1986, a French toxicology journal noted that "Perfumes are increasingly used in an ever wider variety of fields, including perfumes proper, cosmetic products, hygienic products, drugs, detergents and other household products, plastics, industrial greases, oils and solvents, and foods."[4] We can add pesticides to that list. If we include toluene, a sweet-smelling organic solvent, we can also add furniture wax, tires, plastic garbage bags, inks, hair gel, and hairspray.[5]

Perfumes may produce toxic and (more often) allergic respiratory disorders (asthma), as well as neurological and cutaneous disorders.

Numerous federal and state agencies have reported on the

carcinogenic and respiratory toxicity of perfumes and fragrances. In 1986 the *American Journal of Medicine* reported that 72 percent of asthma patients have adverse reactions to perfumes — that is, pulmonary function tests from anywhere between 18 and 58 percent below baseline.[6]

Until the twentieth century, perfumes were made from plants. Now, according to the National Academy of Sciences, 95 percent of them are derived from petroleum and a large number cause cancer, are neurotoxic, are asthmagenic, and irritate the eyes and skin.[3] Indeed, 1,4-dichlorobenzene is a suspected carcinogen, it's a skin and respiratory irritant, and it causes liver and kidney damage, according to OSHA. Despite this, in addition to serving as a pesticide for moths and ants, it's used as a restroom deodorizer.[7,8,]

The EPA has investigated the ingredients in the following classes of popular products: colognes, spray mists, hairsprays, bar soaps, air fresheners, fabric softeners, deodorants/antiperspirants, skin lotions, and nail enamel removers. Ninety percent of the items on the EPA's hazardous waste list was identified in these chemically scented products.[9]

Several hundred ingredients may be found in a single perfume. Even a partial list of these chemicals reads like the contents of a toxic waste site. *Cyclohexanol, galaxolide, methyl ethyl ketone, linalool, benzyl salicylate, vertenex, geraniol, coumarin, musk ketone,* and *musk ambrette* are the ingredients of one perfume. Let's take a look at the last two in this short list: musk ketone and musk ambrette.

During a year when such data were recorded, 1987, musk aroma reportedly accounted for 5 percent of the volume of fragrances sold and 10 percent of their monetary value. A total of seven thousand tons of various musk aromatics were used in fragrances. The three most commonly used musks are the aromatic chemicals musk ambrette, musk ketone, and *musk xylene.*

The problem? Musk scents are neurotoxic.[3] And according to the NAS, there is virtually no testing for the neurotoxic effects of fragrance chemicals.

What makes something neurotoxic? A substance is a neurotoxin when it negatively affects the nervous system. Research published by the NAS tells us that musk ambrette causes central and peripheral nervous system damage. Other aromatics have been found to irritate the upper respiratory tract and depress the immune system. Do you wear a lot of perfume and get sick more than you should?

The NAS states that fragrances should be included in the same category as heavy metals, certain air pollutants, *food additives,* solvents, and *insecticides.* This is some serious company.

The perfume ingredient *cyclohexanol,* has a narcotic effect when it is inhaled. Its MSDA states that it is harmful by inhalation, ingestion, or skin absorption. It is a severe skin and eye irritant.

Aroma-chemicals are not the only perfume ingredients capable of causing a wide variety of health problems. A number of natural biological byproducts are used as well, and hypersensitive people can be expected to react adversely to them. These are essential oils such as civet, galbanum, patchouli oil, asafetida, and bergamot oil. The latter is classified as a hazardous substance and a strong sensitizer on the same order as formaldehyde.

The oil comes from the fruit of a tree that originated in Southeast Asia and now finds a home in Italy. Its citrus fruit has been highly touted for years as an antidepressant with numerous other claimed benefits. It is present in one-third of the world's perfumes. The MSDS states that if the scented oil is inhaled, the victim should be removed to fresh air. Avoidance of skin contact is also recommended.

Here, we need to make a distinction between the strong inhalation of a perfume and a low-dose exposure over time. They are two different phenomena and may have different effects, though both sets of effects may be profound. Short-term exposure to a high dose may lead to an immediate headache, eye and throat irritation (similar to formaldehyde exposure) and mood swings. Long-term exposure may lead to fatigue, ill feeling, sleeplessness in some persons or even drowsiness in others.

Because bergamot oil has a fruity citrus odor, asthmatics should be advised to avoid products in which it is present.

At one time, virtually all department stores added fragrance to their envelopes and bills. It is still a problem. Not only do we get to smell it, but it is also in the glue that we lick to seal the envelope. You may recall that the postal service had flavored stamps for a number of years. Then they listened to complaints and developed the self-adhesive stamp.

One department store used to send their bills with an advertisement written on the envelope for "the only fragrances with a synthesized human pheromone component which promotes attractiveness by enhancing the way we feel about ourselves and how others respond to us."

Pheromones are *sexual attractants* produced by animals and insects. In theory the stores claim sounds fine, but pheromones' presence in humans and the way we perceive them is questionable.

Many national catalogue companies stopped using fragrance in mailings a few years ago, after public pressure forced them to do so.

Many magazines for adults, teenagers, and younger children contain fragrance strips as a form of advertising. These strips are prepared by dipping a paper strip into scented oil so that an odor is emitted. One monthly magazine recently sent me a free issue that contained nine different scent strips.

Scratch and sniff is another form of scented product whose use is self-explanatory. Here, the scent is enclosed in minute capsules. This is widely used in advertising to capture the scent of a new car or rubber tire, lumber, burnt match, flower, mushroom, ham, ketchup, butter, mildew, and detergents.[10]

Fragrances in general are unregulated and untested and have from one to numerous toxic components. It's okay to say no to department store employees who want to spray you with the latest perfume.

Chapter 3
Starting the Day

Before we shampoo and take the morning shower, we must first turn on the water. The problem begins here. Many municipal water districts inject chloramines into the water supply, instead of chlorine. The chloramines react with cells, whether they are bacterial or human. In contact with organic matter, such as human cells, they cause the formation of trihalomethanes.

Data suggest that chlorine alone has the potential of causing damage to human health, but data also tells us that chlorine alone has a thousand-fold or more effect on bacteria in our water supply when compared with the addition of chloramines.

Concerned citizens and the EPA are at odds regarding the use of chloramines in our water supplies.

(Reduction in the level of chlorine and its gases can be reduced if the shower water is cooler to prevent outgassing of the chemical, and the shower times are reduced in length. Operation of the bathroom fan can also help in the escape of the gases.)

I believe that there is a tradeoff. Politics and cost are always involved, but the risk of the public at large being exposed to cholera, E. coli, or *Salmonella* in our water supply must be minimized. Until we can find a better solution or a compromise, what is in place is what gives us a safe water supply—pesticides not withstanding.

Now that the water is on, we can shampoo. A popular *shampoo* for women has twenty-two chemicals plus fragrance. Another brand contains as many as forty ingredients. The male version has somewhat fewer ingredients, plus fragrance. *Hair conditioner* for men has around twelve ingredients plus fragrance.

The typical bar soap will have as many as eighteen ingredients plus fragrance. The fragrances in bar soap and shampoo become volatile (airborne), which means we inhale them in the shower. The effect is enhanced by the *chloroform* and smell of chlorine that comes from the warm water tap.

We dry our heads and bodies with towels that have been washed in laundry detergent with fragrance and a little chlorine *bleach*, then placed in the dryer with an antistatic product plus fragrance.

Skin care lotion has twenty-four ingredients plus perfume. A popular self-action *tanning lotion* has thirty-four ingredients.

After showering, most people use *deodorant* containing about ten ingredients plus fragrance.

Hairspray has eighteen ingredients plus a fragrance and a propellant. Hairspray also has *acrylate* copolymer thickening agent which is a form of plastic.

Isobutane is a common propellant in hair sprays and spray mouth fresheners, non stick cooking sprays, and numerous other products. It is a small hydrocarbon molecule that is liquefied under pressure and becomes a gas when the pressure is released. Isobutane is considered innocuous in terms of causing any health effects when it is used as a carrier propellant for products used in the home. Unless carbon dioxide is used, propellants 'should be considered flammable and should not be used near an open flame.

Many people use body lotion or body talc after the shower. Men use aftershave. Virtually all of these are scented. Makeup frequently contains formaldehyde, and the allergic reactions it causes are well documented.

Toothpaste may contain ten ingredients and a "flavor enhancer." Mouthwash can have twelve ingredients plus "flavor."

It's easy to see how our lungs, hair, skin, and clothing come in contact with an ocean of solvents, dyes, and *chelating agents* to bind the ingredients, perfumes, *emulsifiers*, and various enhancers.

We can be exposed to as many as a hundred or more chemicals and a half-dozen fragrances, and we're not even out of the bathroom yet!

Are we involved in something that is bigger than we are in terms of our exposure to chemical compounds? Are we losing the war for better respiratory health because somebody else is telling us what is good for us and selling us something we don't need? Are we blaming pollen for our breathing problems when the answer is in our bathroom?

Not all chemicals or scented products are bad. In many cases there might even be an improvement over products of past years. If you have concerns about the issue, it might not hurt to stop using certain products altogether. After all, if you don't like what's on TV, you do have a choice—you can turn it off.

In today's world, many products are available that are fragrance free. These include laundry detergents and soaps, skin lotions, and deodorants. The purposeful use of fragrance should be avoided.

Chapter 4

Aromatherapy

Aromatherapy—the use of fragrances and scents to cure a wide variety of physical and mental ailments—is an ongoing science that is thousands of years old. At one time or another, aromatherapy has been touted as a cure for stretch marks and wrinkles, and an effective antidepressant, sedative, or stimulant, depending on the fragrance in question. Whether it can accomplish any of these things will probably be debated for some time, but there is more to talk about in terms of potential respiratory problems.

Why respiratory? *Pinenes* are oils present in pine, nutmeg, and black pepper. They belong to a class of chemicals called *terpenes*. Historically, pine oil has been recommended as a treatment for sore throats, respiratory weakness, various common infections, and the relief of stress.

Another terpene is limonene, present in the citrus fruit known as bergamot. It is also the main constituent in many other *citrus oils*, including *lime, lemon,* and *orange.* It has been recommended as a stimulant to the immune system, a treatment for *herpes,* and a stress reducer.

Both pinenes and *limonenes* have antimicrobial properties. As you might expect, they smell like pine and citrus. Does this mean that they are safe to inhale? Not necessarily. No matter how pleasant or natural something may smell, it can still trigger an asthmatic attack in someone prone to asthma.

Also of concern are the results of a joint study conducted by the University of California, Berkeley, Lawrence Berkeley

National Laboratory, the University of Denmark, and other fa-
cilities. They found that terpenes may react with ozone to form
a number of toxic compounds, including formaldehyde, a class
A2 carcinogen. Ozone is present outdoors and, of course, is
generated indoors by ozone-producing machines dedicated to
the production of ozone in the air. It is also produced as a byproduct of electrically operated office machines such as copiers
and printers. It would seem that purchase of an ozone-generating machine coupled with an air freshener in the room of
an infant, a child, an elderly citizen, or any person concerned
about respiratory health should be reconsidered.[11]

The methods of choice for aromatherapy are bath, com-
press, massage, or *diffuser*. (A diffuser is a device that spreads
the scent of essential oils into the air without the inconvenience
of burning them.) As natural as these fragrances and methods
of application might be, people with chemical sensitivities cannot tolerate them.

Fragrances can be considered respiratory irritants, In that
regard, they are similar to formaldehyde, spices, onion, garlic,
and other food and chemical odors and can have an adverse effect on asthma patients, if not the public at large. Therefore, it is
interesting that, historically, the herbs recommended for treatment of asthma have included cajeput, cypress, eucalyptus,
frankincense, hyssop, lavender, lime, myrrh, spearmint, and
spruce. These plant scents have been used for ages to lessen
symptoms of asthma in various preparations such as lotions
with an oil base, sprays, aqueous solutions, incense, and candles. The leaves and flowers have been added to foods. This is
contrary to today's practice of avoidance.

Modern doctors tell us that many of these treatments will

work to some extent with the right patient at the right time. However, because some 85 percent of asthma is allergy-related, aromatherapy may be a problem for many patients with allergies, whether the herbs or spices are burned, inhaled, or eaten.

Virtually all manner of paper products, soaps, and personal care items are fragranced these days. We are exposed to fragrance strips in magazines and through advertisements that are mailed to us. We even get sprayed as we enter some department stores, though this is becoming less frequent due to awareness of allergies.

Is it only those who are clearly allergic who should be concerned, though? Government agencies and private investigations have found that many of the components of fragrance products, including perfumes, are hazardous to our health via many mechanisms, including absorption, inhalation, and ingestion (of particular concern with scented lip balms and flavored mouthwashes). Our exposure to so many scented items can affect our attitudes and behavior, as noted later in this volume. On a better note, in the non asthmatic person, cinnamon, peppermint, and spearmint may increase alertness for those who might be getting drowsy.

Whether or not the reader is aware of any sensitivity to fragrances and perfumes, it is less irritating to the respiratory tract to avoid contact with these substances as much as possible. Buy fragrance-free soaps, detergents, cosmetics, and paper products. Recycled paper products, for example, are usually fragrance-free and are easy to spot as they are generally brown in color.

Common Lung Irritants

Let's look at the chemicals in some household products that have been around for awhile and that aren't so safe. First, some definitions:

Emulsifiers keep substances together in solution that might normally separate, such as water and oil.

Petroleum distillates (including mineral spirits) are colorless solvents obtained from the distillation of petroleum. They can be highly toxic when a high concentration is inhaled over a short period of time, or a relatively lower concentration is inhaled over a longer period of time. These are flammable and serve as good grease cutters.

Surfactants lower the surface tension of liquids to allow for better penetration. These are used for cleaning purposes.

Dishwasher detergents are powders made of strong alkalis and phosphates (or sodium carbonate, otherwise known as washing soda). Frequently, they contain bleaches, perfumes, colorings, and inactive filling ingredients. These are called fillers. The entire mix not only clears away the grease from dishes, but also prevents them from spotting. Their greatest user hazard comes from inhaling the powder dust when the soap is put into the dishwasher. Liquid soaps might be preferable. In general, however, this is not considered to be a health issue.

Dust control sprays are comprised mostly of *mineral oil*, alcohol, petroleum distillates, surfactant (to dissolve grease), fragrance, and propellant. If you like air fresheners you should love these sprays. The petroleum distillates and fragrances are respiratory irritants and volatile organic compounds that readily enter the airways to become circulated throughout the rooms of the building.

There are new products on the market that address these problems. One of them (Endust) was created specifically without fragrance or petroleum distillates, and has a spray that is designed to be well-directed in order to avoid aerosolization.

Fabric softening sheets are nonwoven sheets of rayon fibers saturated with surfactants and perfume. These work as moisturizers to prevent buildup of static electricity in the clothing. The perfumes can be irritating to the eyes, nose, and throat and cause headaches and dizziness in people exposed to them, even for a short period. They are also absorbed into the clothing and bedding. The use of fragranced antistatic sheets with a fragranced laundry detergent is a potent combination of respiratory irritants.

Furniture polishes contain water, petroleum distillate, emulsifier, wax, and sometimes fragrance. Adequate ventilation is the key to avoid getting into trouble with these products. Polishing furniture may require cross-ventilation in the home to avoid buildup of vapors from these products and to protect the lungs of children and pets.

Mothproofing products with *paradichlorobenzene* are less toxic than those with *naphthalene,* but overexposure to either can cause dizziness.[7] Try to air out clothing the night before wearing it to minimize skin contact with these chemical irritants.

Varnishes commonly contain linseed oil or castor oil, drying agents, and petroleum distillate. Similar to furniture polishes, these products are frequently used over large surface areas.

There should be adequate fresh air ventilation to prevent irritation of the eyes and lungs.

Don't forget to properly dispose of any rags you use, as they are flammable. If stored indoors these rags will be not only a fire hazard, but also an annoying and irritating source of odor, long after the varnish or polish on the furniture dries.

Chapter 6

Air Fresheners

Air fresheners contain essential oils and aromatic chemicals. Many also contain formaldehyde, perfume, and insecticide. Some can decompose into chlorine and phosgene. Their function is to cover up odor; they do not remove them. If you are serious about fresh air, then don't use air fresheners.

Air fresheners are big business. They come in solid, wick (liquid), spray, and plug-in styles. They are available in a wide variety of scents and are used in public and private restrooms, gyms, restaurants, bars, and cars. Usually, air fresheners will contain essential oils and aromatic chemicals or water and propellant. Constituents can include *naphthalene* (banned as a moth repellent due to its carcinogenic properties), phenol, cresol, *methylene chloride*, paradichlorobenzene (p-DCB), ethanol, xylene, and formaldehyde (a carcinogen). At the minimum they will contain a perfume-masking agent.[11]

According to the National Institute for Occupational Safety and Health (NIOSH) and other sources, phenol is an eye, nose, and throat irritant with a sweet, pungent odor. *Cresol* has a similar odor and affects the central nervous system.[7]

Some air fresheners contain *methylene chloride*, a paint stripper and carcinogen. NIOSH describes it as having a chloroform-like odor, and it is an eye and respiratory irritant at higher concentrations. Air fresheners also commonly contain p-DCB, another carcinogen that smells like mothballs.[7,8]

p-DCB is most common in solid and aerosol air fresheners. It is used as a *fumigant, insecticide,* and *germicide*. Similar to ozone, both methylene chloride and p-DCB may cover up a smell or affect the nose so that it loses its ability to smell.

Air fresheners are widely advertised, but they serve no real function in our daily lives, and very little research has gone into their effects on health. Information is seriously lacking. There is little or no state or federal regulation regarding what companies can put into a product and sell for home usage. As a result, they do not have to list their ingredients on the labels, and we have no way of knowing which air fresheners are safer than others. In many cases, even the added fragrance is unregulated and untested, in keeping with the practice of the related perfume and fragrance industry.

Perhaps a rating system should be instituted so the public can decide which air freshener has the least toxicity.

What about the essential oils—concentrated oily substances extracted from plants—that are used in perfumes, antiseptics and antibiotics? Most of us are familiar with the scent of eucalyptus or menthol to clear up congestion. No prescription is required to purchase these, as they are readily available in most health food stores. This may change in the near future.

The smell of essential oils is not recommended for asthmatics or people who are sensitive to chemicals.

Essential oils have a complex chemistry. They contain ingredients such as *terpenes, esters, alcohols, phenols, aldehydes, vitamins,* and *hormones,* such as an *estrogen* found in *sage.* This latter is not recommended for people who are trying to avoid estrogen-like chemicals.

The use of essential oils in air fresheners is questionable. *Natural* essential oils come from plant sources and smell like the plant. Lemon is one example. Artificial oils or perfume oils are made from petrochemicals and have a similar odor to their natural counterparts. The synthetics may act in combination with the other ingredients and have a negative effect on respiratory health.

In 2004, the British Broadcasting Company reported on a study that found that in homes where air fresheners—including sticks, sprays, and aerosols—were used, babies had a higher incidence of diarrhea and mothers had more headaches and depression.[12]

Instead of covering up household odors, get rid of them at their source: Place a half cup of borax in the bottom of the garbage can, grind a lemon peel in the garbage disposal, run the bathroom and kitchen fans more often, check the refrigerator, and discard rotten food, moldy cheese, and fermented jams and jellies. Better fans in public restrooms would be a good substitute for air fresheners.

Airing out the home on a regular basis is one way to provide fresh air without trying to create it.

If you like fragrance in the form of natural scents, then fresh flowers, pine, and herbs such as spearmint are readily available in the marketplace. If you chose to purchase a fragrance product, first make sure you don't react to it before you bring it into the home. For example, allergists tell us that pine is a trigger for asthma.

The off-gassing of the chemicals from air fresheners occurs at very low concentrations. This does not make them safe, however. It just means that their effect on our health is unknown. Low concentration is no excuse for the use of chemicals in a product that is sold in tens of millions of units each year.

It is necessary to understand that combination effects are not only possible, but likely. This means that the effect on the human body can be two to more than one thousand times greater than when one chemical alone is present. This is known as synergism. (Please refer to the chapter What is Synergism?)

When manufacturers include fragrance in the formulation of a product, it is there for us to inhale., As end product users, as consumers, we never realize the potential for harm that might ensue. We inhale the sweetness of the perfume and never realize that we are inhaling a poison. The sweet or perfumed scent should be a clue and a measure of what we are inhaling. Watch for attitudinal and behavior changes, headaches, and effects on your sleep as some of the symptoms of exposure.to these chemicals.

If you are interested in finding out which chemicals are in which common products, Wallace provides a detailed listing in Sweet Poison: The Dangers of Perfume.[13]

Don't be fooled into thinking that a pesticide is harmless to humans just because it is used against insects. Sometimes pesticides are fragranced for indoor usage against insects and sometimes chemicals used in fragrances also double as pesticides. What's up with that? Always follow the cautions given on the label.

Chapter 7

Hazards of Cosmetology

An important, if not necessary part of many lives is the patronage of hair salons, beauty salons, and their supply stores. According to Professional Beauty Association, the beauty industry was worth 38.5 billion dollars in 2006.[14] The beauty business has not only played a role in the lives of women since recorded time, but is becoming a part of men's lives as well.

To accept these salons is to accept their odors. The chemicals that cause these odors have come under scrutiny over the past couple of decades. Where once we accepted them as almost natural, we now examine them from the standpoint of health, not only for the people who handle and breathe them as a part of their careers, but for the public at large.

Numerous medical reports have appeared over the years regarding the hazards of chemicals used in cosmetology. They have been published in such respected journals as the *Proceedings of the National Academy of Sciences, Mutagen Research,* and the *Contact Dermatitis Journal.*

Numerous studies, including those of John report the following: Cosmetology, a predominantly female occupation comprising over half a million women in the United States, has received little attention to potential adverse reproductive outcomes. Cosmetologists (also called hairdressers, stylists, or beauticians) have daily contact with cosmetic products and thus are routinely exposed through inhalation or skin absorption to a wide range of chemicals, including established toxins such as dyes and solvents. Exposure to chemical during pregnancy has been associated with increased spontaneous abortion risk in various occupations.[15]

According to the article, cosmetologists are exposed to a wide range of chemicals, both by skin contact and by inhalation. These include two thousand chemicals, including those in soaps, foaming detergents, dyes, shampoos, rinses, conditioners, bleaches, estrogens, vitamins, suntan products, deodorants, *depilatories* and *hair straighteners*, *nail builders* (hardeners, enamels), propellants, and preservatives.

The chemicals include azo dyes, formaldehyde, heavy metal oxides, and sulfides. Many of these chemicals are not mutagens as such, but are transformed into mutagens in the body. In particular, many chemicals in hair dye are mutagenic, and some cause cancer in laboratory mammals. Certainly, skin disorders and allergies are commonplace and well documented among cosmetologists[16] and links have been found between cosmetologists using their products and a higher frequency of miscarriage, learning disabilities, and behavior disorders among them.[17]

Many pages have been written relating to the subject of exposure of cosmetologists to toxic chemicals. In terms of mutagenic effect and cancer, it must be stressed that the long-term effects of exposure to these chemicals is a big unknown.

The *Journal of Toxicology and Environmental Health* and other journals have presented several reports indicating that cosmetologists were at twice the risk of exposure to direct-acting mutagens compared with dental workers.[15,17] To their credit, many hair salons are now using carbon filtration air purifiers to remove odors from the workplace. Whether this helps prevent development of multiple chemical sensitivity (MCS) in employees and the public at large is be yet to be proved.

Chapter 8

Chemical Sensitivity

In this petrochemical age, imagine not being able to tolerate any fragrance or cleaning agent other than water and a few rare eco-friendly products. Imagine becoming ill with virtually every conceivable symptom, except those caused by microbial attack. Finally, try tending to your clinical reactions with no money, as you have spent it all on doctors who could find nothing wrong, except to tell you that you are depressed. Indeed, people who have true multiple chemical sensitivity (MCS) cannot pick up this book to read it. This is the dilemma that many find themselves in as they become reactive to the petrochemicals that we are sold and to which they are exposed, with no choice about it.

There is a difference between chemical intolerance and chemical sensitivity. A person may not like a particular odor on a personal level. Another person may get a dry throat and itching eyes inside a new manufactured home. And a third person may develop long-lasting symptoms to a wide variety of chemicals if they are exposed to formaldehyde or fragrances or pesticides for a long period of time.

MCS is a form of environmental illness (EI). EI can result from chemical injuries and can be reactivated by subsequent exposure even to low-level amounts of certain chemicals, including fragranced products, glues, solvents, new building materials, inks and a seemingly endless list of product categories. The people with MCS know that the term natural has a broad range of meanings that are not helpful to their cause, and an unscented product may contain masking fragrances that may make the product more toxic to them.

I have worked with MCS sufferers for years and find that they have a vast knowledge about what items or products in our daily lives have which chemicals. Avoidance is their biggest challenge, since our environment is saturated with agents that can trigger a response. Their sensitivity is greater than any instrumentation can measure, which brings the credibility issue into play.

The National Foundation for the Chemically Hypersensitive, and the NCEHS, interviewed 6,800 sufferers. Half reported that their illness began with pesticide exposure. In addition, they report that 11 percent of Americans report sensitivity to chemicals. Up to 4 percent of the U.S. population is chronically ill with CS based on state and federal studies, and 3 percent of Californians report electrical sensitivities.[18]

In 2001, deFrance reported that 12 to 30 percent of the general population has a chemical sensitivity. This sensitivity is due to inflammation related to nerves in the skin and mucous membrane of the airway, gut, and genitourinary tract.[19]

In their acclaimed landmark book, *Chemical Exposures: Low Levels and High Stakes*, Ashford and Miller describe how low-level chemical exposures may cause fatigue, memory impairment, headaches, mood changes, breathing difficulties, and digestive problems, along with a host of other health-related issues. The book identifies four major groups of people with hypersensitivity to low levels of chemicals: individuals with random and unique exposure to various chemicals, occupants of tight buildings, industrial workers who handle chemicals, and residents of communities exposed to toxic chemicals.[20]

Many readers are familiar with persons who are sensitive to chemicals in one guise or another. A variety of national and local agencies are available to assist those who have CS or MCS and want more information. Their information data base is extensive regarding fragrances, perfumes, and a wide variety of petrochemical products that we buy or are submitted to in our daily lives.[21,22]

Fortunately, a number of household cleaning products that can be safely used in the homes of MCS patients are available and they are inexpensive. These include microfiber cloths and mops for dusting; vinegar and lemon (almost universally available, for those who are able to tolerate those smells), baking soda, borax, and fragrance-free degreasers for sinks and showers. (Please see the section on Safe Household Cleaning.)

Endnotes

1. Lavabre, M. 1990. *Aromatherapy Workbook.* Healing Arts Press, Rochester

2. Shehata, M. 2004. *History of Inhalation Therapy.* Alexandria University, Alexandria, Egypt. e-mail: mshehata@yahoo.com.

3. National Academy of Sciences. 1986. *Neurotoxins: At Home and the Workplace.* Report by the Committee on Science and Technology. U.S. House of Representatives. Sept, 16 [Report 99-827]

4. Kendall, J. 1986. Making Sense of Scents. *Ann Dermatol Vernereol,* 113:1,31-41

5. *Shim* C., M.D. and M.H. *Williams,* Jr., M.D. 1986. Affects of Odors in Asthma. *Amer J Med* January, Vol. 80

6. Ibid.

7. NIOSH. *Handbook to Chemical Hazards.* Centers for Disease Control and Prevention. U.S. Department of Health and Human Services. http://www.cdc.gov/niosh/homepage.html

8. Aerotech P&K Laboratories. *Chemical Guide to Indoor Air Quality.* http://www.emlab.com.

9. Wallace, L., E.W. Nelson, and E. Pellizzari. U.S. EPA *Identification of Polar Organic Compounds in Consumer Producers and Common Microenvironments.* Paper #A312 presented at the Annual Meeting of the AWMA.

10. Advameg Inc. 2007. *How Products are Made. Scratch and Sniff: Background, History, Raw Materials,* Manufacturing. Vol. 3 www.madehow.com/volume-3/Scratch-and-Sniff.html.

11. Science Daily. 2006. *Many Cleaners, Air Fresheners May Pose Health Risks When Used Indoors.* May 24 http://www.sciencedaily.com/releases/2006/05/060524123900.htm

12. BBC News. 2004. Report of Air Fresheners and Aerosols Harm Mothers and Children. *Our Toxic Times.* Chemical Injury Information Network, Great Falls. October 19.

13. EcoMall. Sweet Poison: The Dangers of Perfume. Excerpts from

Health Hazard Information. By L. Wallace , EPA http://www.ecomall.com/greenshopping/fragrance.htm.

14. Grindy, B. 2008. National Profile of the Salon Industry. Looking at the Economy Through Beauty-Tinted Lenses. *Professional Beauty Association.*

15. John, E.M. et al. Spontaneous Abortions among Cosmetologists. Dept. of Epidemiology School of Public Health, University of North Carolina.Epid*emiology,* 5(4):147-155.

16. Reolofs, C. et al. 2008. Results from a Community-based Occupational Health Survey of Vietnamese-American Nail Salon Workers. *J. Immigrant Minority Health.* 10(4):553-361.

17, Babish, J.G. et al. 1991. Urinary Mutagens in Cosmetologists and Dental Personnel. *J. Tox. Environ. Health.* 34:197-206.

18. NCEHS National Center for Environmental Health Strategies. Mary Lamielle, Executive Director, 1100 Rural Avenue, Voorhees, NJ. 08043. Ph. 856-429-5350.www.NCEHS.org; marylamielle@ncehs.org

19. deFrance, T. 2001. *The Risk of Neurogenic Inflammation in Chemical Sensitivity,* presented at the 2001 MCS Conference, Santa Fe, New Mexico.

20. Ashford, N.A. and C.S.Miller.1998. *Chemical Exposures: Low Levels and High Stakes.* Wiley Blackwell, Publ. 2nd ed. 464.

21. Ibid.

22. CIIN Chemical Injury Information Network, P.O. Box 301, White Sulphur Springs, MT. 59645. Ph. 406-547-2255. www.CIIN.org.

Section 5

Pesticides and Other Hazards

Pesticides include a wide variety of chemicals and treatment applications. There are at least six hundred different pesticides and fifty thousand different formulations.[1] There are also between 20 and 30 different categories of pesticides As one might suspect, they can be targeted toward the elimination of herbs (weeds), grasses, molds, algae, rodents, insects, and bacteria, as well as other pests.

For many of us, at least 90 percent of our daily cumulative exposure to pesticides occurs at home.[2]

Pesticides applied indoors vaporize from treated surfaces (e.g., carpets and baseboards) and can be re-suspended into the air on particles. Those applied to the foundation or perimeter of a building may penetrate into interior spaces, resulting in measurable indoor air levels. For example, cracks in the slab, which occur commonly, may permit the entry of these agents into the home proper. Pesticides may also be added to carpets, paints, and other furnishings and building materials at the time of manufacture. Consequently, the presence of pesticide residues in indoor air does not necessarily indicate their use within or on the premises.[3]

While occupational inhalation exposure guidelines have been established for many pesticides, the United States has no current guidelines for non occupational indoor air exposures. This means that there are no guidelines for safe levels inside a house, just as there are no guidelines for fragrance products. How does one even begin to know which pesticides and how much of each pesticide is present? There is no answer to that; each of us must undertake our own precautions.

Chapter 1
Pesticides

General information

Pesticides are sold as sprays, liquids, sticks, powders, crystals, balls, and foggers.

Pesticides and herbicides have long been used for bug and weed control at home, school, the workplace, roadways, agriculture, and communitywide applications. The sale of pesticides for lawn care products alone is a large industry, and in many cases their use is justified.

We are mostly concerned with organic pesticides, and not those of a basic inorganic nature such as boric acid or copper sulfate. Organic pesticides are comprised of two primary components. The first is the active ingredient. This kills or retards the growth of a particular group of bugs or weeds. The second component consists of other substances. Listed as "inerts," they make up eighty to 99 percent of the chemical formulation; most are over 95 percent. You can ascertain this by reading the label. Inerts include solvents, stabilizers, emulsifiers, and preservatives; usually in a water base. They are listed as inerts because they do not play an active role in killing the targeted insect or weed; however, their danger to humans is another story.[4]

There are over fifty thousand pesticide products on the market today, and the most common inert ingredients include naphthalene, xylene, toluene, glycol ether, trichloroethane, and dioxin. Recognize any of these names? Inerts are virtually unregulated by the EPA.

In 2008, according to the EPA, a number of investigations throughout the country found that most homes studied contained up to a dozen different pesticides indoors.[5] Furthermore, many of the pesticides identified had never been used in that particular house. This tells us that they are tracked in as part of dust on our shoes or blown in on wind currents.

Pesticides most commonly found in the home included *heptachlor, chlorpyrifos, aldrin, DDT, chlordane, diazinon, atrazine, dieldrin,* and *carbaryl.*

Researchers commonly find that the level of indoor pesticides is ten times or higher indoors than outdoors. This includes pesticides approved for outdoor usage only. Their presence is due to a number of factors: They're sprayed. They're tracked inside on shoes. Stored household pesticide containers are improperly sealed. The outdoor types are exposed to warmer air, evaporate, and enter the home as a gas, which then bind with the dust in protected areas away from sunlight. It is accepted among researchers that when the latter occurs, the pesticides can remain indoors for years, if not decades. Following the behavior of volatile organic compounds in general, we can expect that household surfaces collect and then release the pesticide.[2]

To make matters more interesting, when a pesticide chemical is used in some other function, say, as a room deodorizer, it does not have to be listed on the label of the product. Paradichlorobenzene, for example, is used in air fresheners. This chemical is not only highly toxic to people described as chemically sensitive, but it also seriously affects others to the extent that it may contribute to their eventual sensitivity to chemicals.[6,7,8]

Airborne pesticides

According to the EPA, nearly 90 percent of all households in the U.S. use pesticides. Some 85 percent of the total daily exposure of adults to airborne pesticides comes from breathing air in the home.

Let's take benzene as an example. Nearly 85 percent of atmospheric benzene is produced by cars burning gasoline; the remaining 15 percent is produced by industry.

Nearly all our exposure to benzene is from indoor sources. This is because indoor smoking traps the chemical in the dust, and outdoor dust that contains benzene is tracked indoors. That makes for a compelling reason to take shoes off at the door before entering the home.

In addition, a number of products used indoors contain benzene or related chemicals, including paints and fragrance products in general.

Avoiding the use of mothballs and air fresheners with p-dichlorobenzene reduces the risk of cancer. Avoiding storage of gasoline and lawnmowers in attached garages means less risk of fire and of cancer from benzene.

Dieldrin, a termiticide, was commonly used in the 1970s. Today it is still found in homes, where it is protected from photo-degradation by the sun or wash-out through rainfall. This is also true of chlordane and the major constituent of its formulation, heptachlor.

EPA reports available through the mail or online state that the pesticide pentachlorophenol is so widespread that it was found in the urine of 72 percent of the population tested. Vapors from the active ingredients in Dursban, chlorpyrifos, chlordane, and PCP enter the respiratory system at a much greater rate than the dust particles they have attached to.

Pesticides for outdoor use include insecticides, fungicides, herbicides, rodenticides, termiticides, and mildewcides.

Indoors, nobody knows how much exposure to pesticides is bad for us, as long-term studies are not in agreement.

What does all this mean? Pesticides on the lawn and treatments for bugs and termites in the garden and around the home result in the presence of these chemicals indoors where they can remain from months to decades. Reasons for their relative longevity indoors depends on a number of factors: They are degraded by direct sunlight but last longer under conditions of higher humidity. They can attach to dust particles, but good filtration can reduce the number of these particles. They enter the home through tracking, so removing the shoes at the door will reduce this problem. Fresh air replenishment into the home will result in the expulsion of the product to the outdoors. Mopping baseboards, entries, and exits to the home will remove much of the active agent, if that is so desired.

In some cases, removal of pesticides from the skin and the home is sometimes difficult because many of them are oil-based, not water-based. Part of this exposure comes from direct contact through the users attempt to apply the via aerosol applications of the product. The use of simple isopropyl alcohol can successfully remove many pesticides from the skin.[7]

Inside the home, they are present when we buy and use aerosols, fogs, sprays, and powders and apply them in corners, edges, floors, and the air. Part of this exposure comes from direct contact through the user's attempt to hand-apply aerosol formulations of a product by saturating a cloth. They are present on vegetables, fruits, grains, meats, and some clothing. For example, pesticides remain when a cotton crop is sprayed to hold down insect infestation and then cotton is made into yarn for clothing.

Any kind of heat causes chemicals in pesticides to become airborne to varying degrees, as they are usually in a liquid solution. Although many, if not most pesticides today are water soluble, the effect is basically the same when heat is added, including warmth from sunlight, central heating, or normal temperature changes. Following normal behavior of other VOCs and aerosols, the pesticides then settle onto colder surfaces such as the outside of appliances, mirrors, and windows. This settling usually occurs at night. As these surfaces warm, the chemicals become airborne again to settle into carpets, furniture, bedding, window coverings, and other soft furnishings.

Pesticide spread

Pesticides and their carrier solvents are spread throughout the home by the ventilation system; they either stay in a gas state or become tied to dust particles, similar to other household VOCs.

Once in the carpet, the pesticides work their way into its backing and the pad underneath. Both act as long-term reservoirs that transfer the pesticide to dust. Pesticides then reenter the air as we vacuum. They also enter through normal processes of evaporation, depending on the heat and *relative humidity* (RH), airflow, and other factors within the dwelling. Older upright vacuum cleaners with poor-quality bags contribute a tremendous amount of dust and its constituents to the air of the home.

Aerosol pesticides are used outdoors and indoors against ants, cockroaches, flying insects, and other pests. You hold the can a number of inches away from the insect and spray. Cautions tell us to avoid breathing or coming in direct contact with the pesticide. Otherwise, eye and skin irritation may result. These sprays come in numerous scents, which should serve as a warning.

As noted by the Maryland Department of Agriculture, "The chance for a pesticide to move off-target as the result of volatilization increases as the air and surface temperatures increase, relative humidity decreases, particle or droplet sizes decrease, and air movement increases."[8]

In summary: tracking, air filtration, amount of usage of indoor pesticides, the presence of soft furnishings, vacuuming procedures, the pesticide carrier solvent that is present in the pesticide, and the amount of indoor relative moisture, sunlight and shade, all contribute to the longevity of pesticide in the home.

Medical

Most susceptible to pesticides are infants, children, pregnant women, the elderly, people taking medication, persons undergoing immunotherapy, and those with impaired organ system functions.

Repeated exposure to low doses of pesticides can cause chronic illness, just as can exposure to high doses over a short period of time.

Alternatives can be good or bad

The United States General Services Administration has established a successful program for integrated pest management for thirty million square feet of government offices. We should do the same for our homes and schools. There are specific nontoxic treatments for specific problems, such as the use of mint or coffee grounds to wage the war against ants, or the use of boric acid against scaled insects.

There is a group of pesticides that works very well against cockroaches, *ants, flies, lice,* mosquitoes, *caterpillars, aphids,* and other insects. Also, they are less toxic than most pesticides, unless you are allergic to the *chrysanthemum* flower, which belongs to the ragweed family. The use of this flower against insects dates back to the early *Persians* and *Chinese*.

The presence of this class of pesticides may explain an allergy mystery. An elevated level of antibodies to ragweed can be found in the bloodstream of many people when ragweed is not in season. It is possible that they have been exposed to the *pyrethrum* class of pesticides. (Airborne particles from the degradation of the ragweed plant may also contribute to ragweed exposure.)

Pyrethrum refers to the dried, powdered flower heads of the plant. Pyrethrin is made from the ingredients in the flower that are active against the insect pest. *Pyrethroid* refers to man-made *pyrethrins*. They are more toxic to insects than the other two.

These three insecticides are less toxic than other pesticides on the market. They are available as a powder, liquid concentrate (in a water base), or aerosol. Aerosols are still dangerous to humans when inhaled to any significant degree. This is especially true when the products are used indoors. The propellant used these days is carbon dioxide, as fluorocarbons were taken off the market.

Breathing these compounds results in their immediate absorption into the bloodstream. This may cause immediate and severe effects to ragweed- sensitive people. Using the liquid or powdered form is much less hazardous.

These insecticides act almost instantly against the nervous system of pests. In contrast, boric acid can take days to act. In order to ensure that these pesticides retain their knock-down power, slower-acting ingredients are added to the mix. If you are going to use these compounds for treatment of *fleas* in your pet, be aware that they can be toxic to cats at small doses. Read the directions carefully.

Manmade synthetic pyrethroids are coming into wider use against termites. The advantage these materials have over chlorpyrifos (now commonly used) from a health standpoint is that they degrade more rapidly in the presence of sunlight. If some of it gets loose, it won't last for months or years, as does chlorpyrifos.

Dogs exposed to the herbicide 2,4-D are up to twice as likely to develop malignant lymphoma (one of many forms of cancer of the white blood cells that can occur at any age and are often marked by lymph nodes that are larger than normal), according to a study by the National Cancer Institute. 2,4-D is in over 1,500 pesticide formulations. [9]

Traces of herbicides have been found in rainwater in twenty-three states, mostly in the Midwest and Northeast. These include *alachlor* and *metalachlor*. Herbicides applied to farmlands can vaporize into the atmosphere and travel airborne for great distances,[10] and lawn care pesticides are readily tracked into the home. Concentrations will be much higher in areas next to their application, such as inside homes and schools.

Summary: How pesticides enter the home

In addition to the above, pesticides enter the premises through other mechanisms:

- » through cracks in the foundation or the slab when the building is constructed.
- » present in the wood that was used to construct the home (creosote, a termiticide).
- » on air currents.
- » from the purchase of furnishings that are treated with pesticides during their manufacture.
- » in the natural cotton fibers that make up materials brought into the home.
- » in the fruits, water, vegetables, grains, meats, fish, cere-

als, milk, and juices that we consume, whether they are fresh, frozen, or canned.

» on our hands (and feces) after we handle pesticide-containing sprays, powders, and granules.

» on the feet and in the fur of pet dogs and cats that walk on and roll in dirt and grass.

» on used gardening tools or other items that have been purchased or borrowed.

» in furniture, mattresses, tampons, swabs, and cotton balls.

The subject of estrogen-mimicking pesticides is complicated because some pesticides to not affect estrogen production directly, but act in concert with other pesticides, such as Dieldren, to produce a huge increase in production of the hormone. Endosulfan is just one example.

Chapter 2

Formaldehyde

Formaldehyde is a simple molecule that is frequently combined with urea, another simple molecule. The resulting complex is a marvel, with numerous properties that fit nicely into modern living. It is present in such a wide variety of everyday products that the list boggles the imagination.

For instance, we use formaldehyde in foam insulation, plywood, chipboard, textiles, plastics, resins, paints, and glues. It is used in the making of shoes and automobiles. It is also found in dyes, adhesives, and leather products.

Modern furniture is frequently constructed of particle board interior with wood veneer on the outer surfaces. Formaldehyde is used in the manufacture of both, although formaldehyde-free products are available. Wallpaper can emit formaldehyde, especially the prepasted types and those consisting of fibers or layers of paper bonded with formaldehyde-containing resins. Add curtains of cellulose acetate and bed sheets. Starch-based glues, room deodorizers, shampoos, and cosmetics can contain urea-formaldehyde (UF) resins. In paper products, it is used to add wetness strength.

Paper products with UF resin include grocery bags, waxed paper, facial tissues, napkins, paper towels, and feminine hygiene products. UF resins are added to fabrics to provide shrink resistance, permanent press capabilities, water repellency, fire-retarding properties, and fixation of color.

Formaldehyde is a common respiratory and eye irritant, and it is carcinogenic in extremely high concentrations. With low doses of everyday exposure, however, the effects of formaldehyde on the human body when inhaled are considered to be minimal to the extent that the effects can't be measured.

Effects of formaldehyde

Formaldehyde is a very soluble chemical. It dissolves in the moist mucous of the nose and throat and rarely penetrates the mucous membranes under normal background conditions. Its odor is pungent, but it dissolves in the body within a minute and a half, where it is turned into carbon dioxide and water. Basically, formaldehyde stays in the upper respiratory tract. The exception occurs when smokers inhale it into the lungs.

Human beings usually begin to smell formaldehyde at about 0.1 to 3.0 parts per million (ppm). Eye irritation follows smell. At the 8 ppm level, it penetrates the mucous lining of the respiratory tract to cause irritation and distress.[11]

There are some unknowns about formaldehyde. For instance, very little is known about its combination with other chemicals and the effects of these combinations on the individual. People who state that they are chemically sensitive will exhibit a variety of nerve and muscle-related symptoms when in the presence of extremely small amounts of this substance. These symptoms include headache, nausea, dizziness, fatigue, disorientation, and loss of short-term memory. The symptoms can last from minutes to days or even longer.

At extremely low concentrations formaldehyde can produce coughing, constriction in the chest, and wheezing. The level of formaldehyde in room air depends on the rate of exchange of air, the area of the emitting surface, the total air volume, and other factors such as humidity, temperature, and age of the source. The amount of the agent to which a person can react depends on the sensitivity of the person and the dosage and length of exposure time.

It is known that formaldehyde is a sensitizer, similar to its close relative glutaraldehyde (used for sterilization of instruments in dentists' offices) and bergamot. This means that exposure to enough formaldehyde can cause the body to become sensitized to other chemicals. The same thing occurs when overexposure to one pollen or mold type sensitizes the body to many pollen and mold types. The difference here is that in one case the body becomes sensitized to chemicals, and in the other the body is sensitized to allergens.

It is important to remember that formaldehyde is readily absorbed by moisture, whether in the air, lungs, nose, eyes, or skin. Heavily debated is the finding that repeated exposure to formaldehyde liquid or vapor can cause certain individuals to become sensitized. Upon re-exposure to formaldehyde or to related substances (and sometimes to apparently nonrelated substances), these persons may exhibit allergic dermatitis or mild to severe asthmatic reactions.

The people most easily and commonly affected by formaldehyde gas are those who already have respiratory vulnerabilities: the elderly, the infirm, and children. According to the National Institute for Occupational Safety and Health, formaldehyde can cause irritated eyes and tearing, burning of the nose and throat, cough, bronchial spasms, pulmonary irritation, dermatitis, nausea, loss of consciousness, vomiting, and possibly cancer.

Formaldehyde in buildings

Exposure to formaldehyde is virtually unavoidable. The energy crisis of the 1970s led to measures for tightening up buildings and reducing the rate of exchange between indoor and outdoor air. (Please refer to chapter on Traveling by Commercial Airplane.) This practice, coupled with "improved" product technology, led to an increase in the indoor air concentration of formaldehyde.

Formaldehyde is present in clothing stores at 0.9 to 3.3 ppm. Smoke from a log-burning fireplace contains a lot more formaldehyde than smoke from non-wood fires.

It is common to blame the smell of new carpets on formaldehyde. However, carpeting manufactured in the United States has not contained formaldehyde for two decades. There is a paucity of information regarding the presence of this agent in carpets made abroad. In any case, the vast majority of these foreign-made carpets are smaller in size and only serve as area rugs and virtually all commercial and domestic wall-to-wall carpeting used in the United States is made here under the auspices of the Carpet and Rug Institute.

In the vast majority of cases, the odor of domestic carpeting is due to other volatile organic compounds present in the adhesives that hold the carpet surface to the backing, the padding, or for industrial carpeting, those that hold the carpet backing to the floor. These odors quickly dissipate under normal conditions where fresh air is allowed.

Formaldehyde is found in most homes at 0.03 ppm, in mobile homes at zero to 2.0 ppm, and in offices and day care centers at 0.4 to 0.6 ppm. Smokers inhale formaldehyde at 5 to 8 ppm, but sidestream smoke contains it at the level of 30 to 40 ppm. It is also emitted from wood-burning fireplaces at low to high concentrations indoors.

In schools, pressed wood and particle board comprises the cabinet structure.

Homes with urea-formaldehyde foam insulation (UFFI) have been found to contain three to twenty times the formaldehyde level as non-UFFI homes, reaching levels of 0.2 ppm and above. However, mobile homes are repeatedly the worst offenders in terms of releasing formaldehyde gas. Here the air concentrations range from 0.1 to 1.0 ppm. Particle board and plywood are the major culprits here, because the counters, cabinets, paneling, and other woodwork in mobile homes are made with formaldehyde as an agent to hold the particles and the pieces together. The paneling in mobile homes is made from a synthetic wood-resin mixture coated with a varnish that will outgas. This outgassing of varnish and underlying formaldehyde will continue indefinitely as long as the doors are closed. A baking soda wash will remove a great deal of the surface chemical emissions. I recommend periodic treatment of the inner cabinetry of mobile homes and newly constructed homes.

The kitchen areas of mobile homes are the worst, followed by the bedroom. In the kitchen, a high percentage of structural material is made of textile products and artificial wood.

The reader may recall the mobile homes that were provided to victims of hurricane Katrina. They could not be occupied because of the high concentration of formaldehyde. The indoor level can reach one-tenth part per million throughout the interior of the structure and a full one part per million in the kitchen area.

If you are concerned about formaldehyde in your home or business, remember that most of the chemicals used indoors outgas from their materials quickly over a period of days to weeks with lots of fresh air. After this, they usually outgas slowly in low amounts for months or years.

Protecting yourself from formaldehyde

Coating or painting a formaldehyde-emitting object is an easy way to retard its emission. A number of commercially available vapor barrier paints are available for this purpose (ask your local paint dealer). As a general rule, it is a good idea to use plenty of ventilation while painting. Use two coats of the vapor barrier paints.

Emission can also be reduced by using Mylar or vinyl wallpaper with a heavy canvas backing. If you suspect medical problems are occurring because some furniture product is emitting formaldehyde, use plenty of open-window fresh air to dilute the gas until you decide what to do.

Ideally, getting rid of the source is best. Because the outgassing rate of formaldehyde depends on temperature and humidity, simply lowering the thermostat and not using a humidifier can significantly reduce emissions.

Has attic or crawlspace insulation been installed within the past few years? It is a good idea to find out exactly what was installed and to have any joints in the attic ductwork inspected for breaks.

There are two types of formaldehyde-based glues: urea-formaldehyde and phenol formaldehyde. Protection against these can be problematic. Their emissions can continue for an extended period of time, as can the emissions from the paints and varnishes they may be coated with, such as within cabinetry.

Unfortunately, today's trend is to construct a home comprised of a shell made out of OSB and plywood, with cabinets comprised of particle board with lots of veneer, all of which make the homes similar to manufactured homes in terms of their construction and the amount of formaldehyde they contain. There is little the homebuyer can do to reduce the amount of this substance in the air, other than coating textile products and giving the new residence plenty of fresh air. I would suggest that the home buyer seek a residence that is twenty to thirty years old and is constructed of brick, adobe, or slump block. Any formaldehyde that might have been present at one time will have outgassed and overall, its presence will be minimized.

For personal care items such as deodorants and hair care products, read the label. For wood products, avoid particle board, chip board, and plywood. Ask questions. Wash new bed sheets before using them.

Some air cleaners claim to have the ability to remove formaldehyde from the air. If they contain activated charcoal, they may or may not be effective. Only specially treated activated charcoal can remove airborne formaldehyde. (See the chapter on air purifiers.)

Source control, ventilation, and filtration are three methods to deal with the formaldehyde problem. In the first case, source control can include a method to seal in the chemicals and prevent their escape into breathing spaces. Commercial sealants are available for these purposes. If not sealed in, formaldehyde and varnish odors are absorbed into plastics, Styrofoam products, and dish towels for an extended period of time. The second method for dealing with an outgassing problem is ventilation. Plenty of outdoor air, not recirculated conditioned air, is the true key to ridding your airspace of unwanted vapors. It won't happen overnight, but it will happen.

The filtration method of gas removal involves a number of methods, including special activated charcoal, volcanic rock particulates (*zeolite*), and some very new, inexpensive, high-tech filters that are available via the Internet or big city companies that create made-to-order filters.

Chapter 3

Sewer Gas

Nearly everyone recognizes the odor of *sewer gas*. How does it get into our buildings, and is it toxic?

Sewer gas is a common term for a complex mixture of chemicals that are formed during the decay or processing of waste. Two common, highly toxic components of sewer gas include hydrogen sulfide and ammonia. In addition, the gas typically contains methane, carbon dioxide, sulfur dioxide, nitrous oxides, and biological agents. Chlorine bleach, cleaners and solvents, and gasoline are frequently present in both municipal and private sewage treatment systems.[12]

The smell of sewer gas means that there is a decomposition of organic debris by bacteria. A number of gases are released by bacterial action and one of them, *hydrogen sulfide*, smells like rotten eggs. Hydrogen sulfide is toxic, given a high enough concentration, which will depend on the individual's sensitivity. The fire department may tell you that it is not toxic. This means that it won't have any lasting effects after you get an abundance of fresh air. But our definition of the word is different than theirs. Burning eyes, coughing, nausea, headaches, disorientation, and sleeplessness mean that the gas is toxic. And in some people, various symptoms may last for prolonged periods.

The nose is our early warning system. We can detect the smell of sewer gas at a concentration of less than one-four hundredth the official toxicity level.[13] The problem here is that hydrogen sulfide fatigues the sense of smell quickly. We are unable to detect the classical rotten egg odor of the gas, or any other odors, before long.

If you find yourself overwhelmed by the odor of this gas, find some fresh air for a few minutes to free the sense of smell once again, and return to the problem area. This should give you a better indication of whether the gas is present or has gone.

All toilets are vented and so is our sewage system. Manhole covers have holes in them, and toilets are vented with pipes that connect the sewage system to the roof. This prevents the buildup of flammable and explosive gases. However, sewer gas can enter buildings in a number of ways. In a commercial setting, the roof vent stacks can be located within feet of an air conditioner that also takes in fresh air. When the wind blows the wrong way, the sewer gas blows into the fresh air intake of the air conditioner, and from there it will be conducted into the building.

This does not happen in homes because the air conditioner recycles all the air with no fresh air makeup. With the air conditioner off, a window open on the leeward side of the home can permit the entry of gas generated on the windward side, possibly originating from a manhole cover in the street or from a sewage treatment plant nearby.

Another way that gas can enter the home is when residents use the fireplace. This creates a need for fresh air to enter, in order to replace that which is consumed, and outdoor air will be drawn through cracks in doors and windows. Creation of negative pressure within a home can also occur when kitchen and bathroom fans are used.

Schools and commercial buildings contain floor drains, built to receive floor water after mopping. These drains lead to the sewage system and have a curved piece of pipe which is known as a P or S trap—a bent pipe that is made to contain a certain amount of water to keep the sewer smell out of the building. After a period of disuse, these traps dry up, after which sewer gas rises into the building. Filling the pipe with water again quickly solves the problem.

In an apartment building, an upper unit occupant may fill and drain the sink. This may cause the water in the lower units to empty water out of the P traps and cause a rotten egg smell in everyone's residence. A dry P trap can also occur in a sink that has not been used for a long time or has been newly repaired, or in a floor drain present in the heater, air conditioner closet, or elsewhere, as noted above.

Additionally, low-lying areas can accumulate the gas. Basements, underground vaults, excavations and pits in proximity to sewer lines, septic systems, landfills, and wetlands/swamps may also accumulate the gas, especially the hydrogen sulfide and methane portions. These are explosive.

Chapter 4

Burning and Other Uses for Tires

Generally, tires contain the same level of heavy metals as coal. The exceptions here are *chromium* and *zinc*. Chromium is present in steel-belted tires and zinc is necessary for the rubber-annealing process.

Chlorine concentrations are also higher in tires than in other fuels.

The issue of what to do with discarded used tires has become a worldwide environmental problem. Only a fraction of them can be used for *asphalt* or road construction. If left in the open, they collect water, and mosquitoes will use them to breed. In addition, they are unsightly and take up space in storage yards and backyards.

One alternative is burning. A huge number of tires are taken out of the environment and burned for energy. The EPA lists one hundred and twelve companies in the United States that burn tires as a sole fuel, or as a fuel supplement added to *coal, coke, fuel oil,* or *natural gas.* These plants burn two hundred to three hundred tires per hour, and 45 percent of the recycled tires are burned.[15] While this keeps the material out of landfills, the tradeoff is increased atmospheric pollution that is often well above state and federal health standards.

When tires are added to another fuel source, the general trend is for carbon monoxide (CO) emissions to increase because of incomplete combustion. CO is a poisonous gas and its large scale release into the atmosphere has generated concerns by citizen's groups. I have served as an expert witness in this matter. (Please refer to chapters on house fires, and candles.) More importantly, along with CO production comes the emission of *dioxins* and *furans*, the most toxic carcinogens known. Dioxins and furans are formed as a result of incomplete combustion in the presence of chlorine. In many cases, the emissions of dioxins and furans have not been monitored adequately for tire burning.

Indeed, the issue of CO emission levels is frequently challenged by those who burn the tires because the number of tires (reported) that are burned in different coal or tire burning plants will vary. In general, about fifty-three million tires per year are consumed as fuel in U.S. cement kilns.[14]

There are a number of possible alternatives to burning, such as development of new technologies that incorporate tire chips, as well as the creation of microscopic tire fragments for construction, waterproofing of clothing, and other materials. Shredded and crumb rubber created from tires are currently being used for athletic field tracks, playgrounds, floor mats, belts, shoe soles, washers, and, as noted above, for cement making.

Chapter 5
Roof and Street Tarring

Hazardous chemicals are released into the air by the process of street or *roof tarring*. These can find their way into the indoor air through cracks in window and *door frames*, or through open doors and windows.

These agents come in two general categories: vapors and particulates.

The vapors primarily consist of volatile organic compounds (VOCs) such as benzene, toluene, sulfur, aldehydes (especially formaldehyde), sulfur dioxide, carbon monoxide, naphtha and kerosene.

The EPA classes the particulates as polycyclic organic matter (POM). These are tiny globules that range in size from less than one micrometer (smaller than a bacterium) to fifty or more micrometers (about the size of a pollen grain). Under the microscope they appear black and spherical, and they consist of the solid state of the above gases in the form of time-release capsules for VOCs. They appear black because they are opaque to light.

Street and roof tarring are necessary in today's society. Street tarring is performed using what is known as cutback asphalts. These fall into the categories of rapid-cure, medium-cure, and slow-cure road oils, depending on the circumstance of use and the area of the country. Cutback asphalts are prepared by blending asphalt cement with heavy oils, kerosene-type solvents, or naphtha (coal tar) and *gasoline* solvents. In fact, the asphalt may contain over a dozen petrochemical ingredients.[16]

No control devices are employed to reduce evaporative emissions from cutback asphalts. Emulsified rapid cure asphalts are used more and more frequently. This involves cutting the oil with detergents, which are added to water, rather than with toxic solvents. Limited test data suggest that from this type of asphalt, 75 percent of the solvent is lost on the first day after application, 90 percent within the first month, and 95 percent in three to four months.

Evaporation takes place more slowly from medium-cure asphalts, with roughly 20 percent of the solvent emitted during the first day, 50 percent during the first week, and 70 percent after three to four months. The evaporation rate is much slower in cooler weather and more rapid in the case of roof tarring, where less material is involved. The odors can carry for several blocks.

Armed with this knowledge you might consider renting a motel room for a day or two if tarring is scheduled in your neighborhood.

Nearby tarring is annoying at best. The VOCs will be emitted for months after application. This is an important consideration when shopping for a new residence if health is your concern. Find out if the roads are scheduled to be tarred or chip-sealed in the near future. If you are chemically sensitive, this is one more factor in your decision to move to this area of town.

Chapter 6
Mixing Bleach with Ammonia

The misuse of household cleaning agents has been reported in a variety of medical-related and housekeeping journals over the years. One common example is the mixture of chlorine bleach with ammonia.

Household bleach contains 5.25 percent sodium hypochlorite. Household ammonia consists of 5 to 10 percent ammonia in water. Separately, these agents have low potential for toxic inhalation injury. If you breathe a combination of the two agents, however, problems can occur, as will be described. Combining them causes the formation of chloramine gases added to our drinking water to kill microorganisms. Chloramines may make us more reactive to all chemicals, similar to the effect of formaldehyde. (See the chapter on Starting the Day.)

When these gases come into contact with the skin and moist body surfaces such as the eyes, nose, and especially the upper respiratory tract, they combine with water molecules to produce hydrochloric acid (HCl) and other acids. These cause tissue irritation. Hydrochloric acid also goes by the name of muriatic acid and is best known for its use in swimming pools. In the pool, chloramines are what cause irritation to swimmers' eyes.

Once the acid or acids are formed in the tissues, a variety of symptoms can result, including cough, hoarseness, sore throat, headache, and tearing of the eyes. In extreme cases, difficulty breathing and shortness of breath may occur for months afterward.

Fortunately, severe exposures rarely develop into *pneumonitis* and related disorders. The amount of irritation depends on the amount of gas produced, the exposure time, and the water content of the exposed tissues. It also depends on the age and relative health of the person at the time of exposure.

Several hundred cases have been reported, with symptoms lasting from one to six hours. Fresh air and cool liquids served as their main therapy. In more severe cases, emergency treatment by paramedics with bronchodilator usage and oxygen is suggested.

Fresh air ventilation of the home is a must to limit further exposure to occupants, including children and pets.

Also, be aware that hydrochloric acid will form in the lungs and outside the body on other moist surfaces in the area where the mixture was created. This could lead to corrosion of stainless steel surfaces, especially on countertops and other household items. Neutralize suspect areas that may have been exposed to the acid with baking soda (one cup in a gallon of warm water) and light buffing with a soft cloth and a nonabrasive polish.

Chapter 7

John and Jane Johnson

As Jane sprays her hair this Saturday morning, she breathes in a dose of aerosol propellant. Borderline asthmatic, Jane has to take time out to catch her breath. John, on the other hand, avoids aerosols. He uses a pump sprayer to add a little musk scent to his body. What John doesn't know is that musk is a toxic product that can affect the nervous system. And it is unregulated, like most perfumes. This means his behavior and attitudes may deteriorate, and the smell may aggravate Jane's asthma. If John had known this, he would have suspected that the information didn't apply to them, anyway, only to everyone else.

John and Jane go shopping. In the clothing store they are greeted with formaldehyde at ten to one hundred times the level above the human detection limit. Formaldehyde is used as a fire retardant in clothing and for permanent press fabrics. Their eyes water, their throats burn, and they cough. They both complain of a spacey feeling.

In the carpet store they are greeted by 4PC, the adhesive that bonds the top of the carpet to the backing.

The supermarket has such a complex mixture of smells: fried chicken, fragranced laundry detergent, bleach, and cleaning products. They buy a little of each and go to a department store. A handy hostess gives them each a spray of perfume.

Their busy schedule calls for a trip to the video store for a couple of the latest scents in plastic—soft plastic outgases more than hard plastic.

John has to make a quick stop at the office. It's closed on Saturday. Three thousand square feet of new carpeting await him. In a move to conserve energy, his employer has opted to keep the amount of fresh air pulled in by the air conditioner to a minimum. Without fresh air, the chemical smell will be distributed throughout the building without being diluted, to greet workers the next Monday morning.

Unaware of the hazards present indoors and believing himself to be a conscientious person, John steps outside to smoke a quick cigarette.

At home, John begins to polish the furniture with commercial polish. The air concentration of petroleum-based volatile organic compounds increases tenfold within minutes. John turns on a central fan, thinking that will help. Jane starts to get a headache.

"Think I'll clean up in the kitchen," says Jane after dinner. With several cleaning agents readily at hand, Jane accidentally knocks the open ammonia container into the bucket of concentrated bleach solution, liberating chlorine and chloramine gases. John calls the paramedics to treat her asthma attack.

Jane is admitted to a hospital, where she is tended to by a bevy of doctors and nurses who wear latex gloves lubricated with cornstarch. The microscopic starch particles cling to their clothing as a fine dust. These particles carry the latex antigen and make one or two of the attendants cough. One of them sneezes. Jane's latex allergy becomes activated and her respiratory condition worsens. The particles are carried in the air throughout the hospital.

Jane is wheeled to X-ray. Here she encounters X-ray photographic development chemicals. These include glutaraldehyde, which sensitizes radiologists to chemicals in general. This is released into the air near a waiting room to affect other patients.

At last Jane is moved to a room. Unfortunately, the pleated filters in the hospital's central air handling unit have recently collapsed from overload. Though they have been changed every three months for years based on manufacturer's recommendations, only nine weeks have passed since they were installed.

Construction is going on at this hospital. Several of the wings are being remodeled, with plastic sheeting holding in the dust. The plastic sheets are not carefully placed, and *Aspergillus* mold spores associated with the dust are released into the air, affecting immunocompromised patients in a wing down the hall. Many of them develop a fungal disease of the lungs and ears.

Jane is released the next day. She and John find their car, which he parked early that morning near the loading dock of the hospital—beneath the first floor, where all the diesel trucks are idling near a sign that says "No Smoking!" The diesel fumes add a fragrance that enters the hospital's air-handling system, also located in the basement. Some fumes waft to the roof of the hospital, where the fresh air intakes and exhaust vents are located in close proximity to each other.

John and Jane get home at last. He decides to mow the lawn. Because it's such a nice day, he opens the doors and windows to air out the house while he operates the power mower. Herbicide-laden grass particles and gas fumes enter the home. John finishes work and comes indoors, taking off his work clothes in the laundry area. He shakes them out before putting them in the washer.

Just another average weekend for the Johnsons. They could hardly wait for the holidays to arrive.

Chapter 8

Cancer-Causing Agents in Our Air and Food

Countless books and articles have been written on the subject of cancer-causing agents.

As discussed in the chapter on pesticides, there are estrogen-like compounds in our environment, some natural and some synthetic. The natural ones are found in foods such as *broccoli, cauliflower*, and *soy* products. These help to reduce the level of one of the two primary forms of the hormone, estrogen. The synthetic ones mimic estrogen and bind to estrogen receptor sites on our cells. This is unwanted because the presence of estrogen has been found to promote the spread of cancer cells. These agents are found in chlordane, DDT, *atrazine*, *methoxychlor, kepone*, plastics, and aromatic hydrocarbons. The latter are components of petroleum and include gasoline, and are found in many, if not most, petroleum distillates used in polishes and cleaners, fragrances, and perfumes.

DDT persists in the environment for more than fifty years. DDT was banned in the U.S. in 1972 as an active ingredient, but used as an "inert" ingredient until the late 1980s. It is still used outside the U.S. as a pesticide and can be found in many imported crops. Its role in the eradication of the malaria-causing mosquito versus its potential harm to the environment still remains a hotly debated issue.

Methoxychlor is an insecticide used on trees and vegetables.

Kepone was used in ant and roach traps until 1977. It can still be identified in our environment, outdoors and indoors.

We have all had direct contact with these pesticides. They are eaten by cattle in their diet of grasses and grains, and stored in their fat. The cattle are eaten by humans, and the insecticides and pesticides are absorbed and stored in human fatty tissue. The pesticides do not degrade well in the body and persist for decades.

The fact that many of these agents are no longer used is irrelevant. Exposure builds up over time. New estrogen-like chemicals are being produced. Furthermore, estrogen-like compounds are released into the air when we overheat plastics.

What can we do? We can educate ourselves regarding our indoor environment, which is the primary goal of this book. We can promote research in the field of safer pesticides. We can avoid eating animal fat because pesticides are stored in the fat. We can wash fruits and vegetables thoroughly, because they are sprayed with pesticides whether they are domestic or foreign grown. We can be extremely cautious of the use of pesticides in and around the home, as they are inhaled, ingested, and absorbed through the skin. We can develop an integrated pest management system for the home and especially our schools.

Endnotes

1. Spengler, J.D., J.M. Samet and J.F. McCarthy. 2001. *Indoor Air Quality Handbook*. McGraw-Hill, New York. Pesticides. 35.1.

2. Ibid. 35.6.

3. Ibid. 35.5.

4. EPA. 2008. *An Introduction to Indoor Air Quality: Pesticides*. November 25. http://www.epa.gov/iaq/pesticid.html.

5. Ibid.

6. Wallace, L. 1989. EPA. Major Sources of Benzene Exposure. *Environ Health Perspectives*. 82:165-169.

7. Province of British Columbia Department of Agriculture and Lands. 2007. *Pesticide Poisoning*. http://www.al.gov.bc.ca/pesticides/g_1.htm.

8. Maryland Department of Agriculture, Pesticide Regulation Section. 2001. *Reducing off-target Movement of Pesticides* Aug 13-15 Indoors. Reported in Our Toxic Times, (newsletter of the Chemical Injury Information Network) Dec 2004. www.mda.state.us.

9. National Cancer Institute. *Non-Hodgkin's Lymphoma*. http://ccr.cancer.gov/resources/cop/non_hodgkins_lymphoma.asp.

10. Global Pesticide Campaigner. 2001. 11(2) http://www.panna.org/legacy/gpc/gpc_200108.11.2.pdf.

11. U.S. Consumer Product Safety Commission. 1997. *An Update on Formaldehyde*. CPSC Document 725. www.cpsc.gov/cpscpub/pubs/725.html.

12. Envirochex. 2008. *Overview of Sewer Gas*. http://www.envirochex.com/Topic_Other/Sewer_Gas.htm.

13. Ibid.

14. Kristoff,S. 2008. *Recycling Used Automobile Tires*. Environmental Engineering. EPA.http://environmental-engineering.suite101.com/article.cfm/recycling_us.gov.

15. EPA. 2008. *Tire Derived Fuel. Scrap Tires.* HTTP://www.epa.gov/epawaste/conserve/materials/tires/tdf.htm.

16. Valero Marketing and Supply Company. *MC Cutback Asphalt.* San Antonio. www.valero.com/NR/rdonlyres/4D14AF0B-8C5A-4CC7-A2C7-60198B3EA296/0/MCCutbackAsphalt211.pdf.

Section 6

Indoor Air Quality

Most people are now familiar with the term "sick building syndrome," or SBS. This term was born in the 1970s, when a need to conserve energy dominated our building and lifestyle habits, resulting in the construction of tighter buildings. This in turn led to an inadequate supply of fresh air to dilute both the indoor pollutants that we brought in and the outgassing of old and new structural materials. The end result was that more people became sick with a variety of new ailments, including chemical sensitivity and an alarming increase in the number of asthma patients. These were just the clinical manifestations. The subclinical symptoms were taking a toll on our quality of life, but couldn't be immediately measured in any scientific sense. Eventually, over the decades, we could measure one thing: time was being taken from our lives. Eventually we found that a reduction of our exposure to particulates of a certain size led to longer life spans.

It is no secret that the rate of cancer and various respiratory diseases has been increasing in the United States.

Scientific American (February 1998) discusses just this issue in an article entitled "Everyday Exposure to Toxic Pollutants."[1] The article points to some sobering facts.

We spend 90 percent of our time indoors, where our exposure to toxins is five to ten times what it would be outside, and for many people, 90 percent of daily cumulative exposure to pesticides occurs at home.[1] Our state and federal governments were once spending virtually all their air-quality money for outdoor air pollution. The level of indoor pesticides is ten times higher than outdoors in virtually every study conducted—including pesticides approved for outdoor usage only.[2]

The average concentration of benzene (present in gasoline and household products, including some paints), and cigarette smoke is three times higher indoors than outdoors.

The authors of the article ask this question: Could everyday items be more of a health threat than industrial pollution, even when homes are surrounded by factories? The answer is yes.

There are two categories of pollutants we should be concerned with regarding our longevity and day-to-day health: particles and gases. As has been shown, both are present indoors, and both can be reduced through simple actions and slight changes in the way we organize our lives. It's called air management. Let's take a closer look at just a few ideas that will save us money and give the entire family better health at the same time.

Chapter 1

General Problems with Gases and Particles

_____

Gases

Gases (vapors) may be present without particles. On the other hand, gases are always present when particles are present; either they are found in between the particles, or the gas molecules are attached to them.

One class of chemical gases is exemplified by carbon monoxide, ammonia, and free chlorine. As free gases they do not attach to particles, per se.

Another class of gases is volatile organic compounds (VOCs). These are chemicals that evaporate readily, which enables us to smell them in most cases. They include acetone in nail polish and polish remover, mold odor, formaldehyde, furniture polish and floor polish, the thousands of products that contain petroleum distillates, hairspray and spray insecticides, hundreds of products that contain fragrance, carpets and their glues, old-style paints that are not eco-friendly, varnishes, and thousands of products that fit into these categories. They also include such harmless smells as brewed coffee and microwave popcorn (containing chemically derived butter). Many of these do attach to dust particles, especially pesticides. This is because dust particles generally maintain a positive charge. That is why electrostatic filters and electronic air cleaners maintain a negative charge across the grid—to attract the particles. When free radicals are formed out of the above list of gases, they can attach to the dust motes. Free radicals can be formed through the action of sunlight or through ozonation. The gases may also adsorb to the surface of the dust particle.

Virtually all of them are lung irritants and will probably make our allergies worse if their level in household air is too high.

Almost every indoor environment will have some background VOCs. These can be measured at a level of 0.1 to 0.3 parts per million, as I have determined over the years. This background level includes coffee; fragrance on clothing that has been washed and dried in fragrance detergent, fabric softener and anti-static products, deodorants and hairspray, natural human odor, and a dozen other scents that we normally encounter in our daily lives.

It is mainly the petroleum-based products that lead to trouble. These include petroleum distillates, pesticides, solvents, and cleaners.

Tetrachloroethylene, the dry-cleaning agent, is a carcinogen. Moth-repellent cakes or crystals, toilet disinfectants, and deodorizers are the major sources of exposure to paradichlorobenzene. Both of these chemicals are carcinogens.

Learn to steer clear of benzene, petroleum distillates, and indoor pesticides, whether they smell like flowers or lemons or they are unscented.

Clinical symptoms of overexposure to VOCs include headache, itching and watering eyes, sore throat, coughing, development of sensitivity to chemicals in general, and even loss of short-term memory. Some symptoms may be temporary and others may be permanent.

Okay, enough with the facts about excess VOCs. Let's talk about how to get rid of them.

The main problem with VOCs indoors is that they build up in concentration because we don't open the home or office to air it out on a regular basis. This is not always possible when prevailing outdoor conditions include high winds that blow dust, frigid temperatures, etc. However, it is still a good practice to do so, even if you can only maintain a small draft for a short period of time throughout the residence.

The indoor VOC level can reach as high as ten to sixty parts per million. This can result from an airtight home or business that does not have enough fresh air. The good news is that in almost all instances, the level of indoor VOCs can be reduced by source removal, such as cessation of the use of petroleum distillates for furniture polishing.

There are several remedies for a reduction in indoor VOC level. Optimally, let fresh air into the home or business and let stale air out as frequently as is practical. Open the windows and doors. Ceiling vent fans (garage) and bathroom fans work well for this purpose. Even weekly air changes in the morning, with tabletop fans or central-air fans, will help reduce the level of VOCs that tend to concentrate in certain areas. Whenever the structure is closed, the VOC level will become elevated again, but each time it will be to a lesser extent.

In more extreme conditions, wash the walls, floors, and cabinets with a solution of one-half cup baking soda in a bucket of warm water. You will have to empty the cabinets before you do this. Change the water in the bucket at least four to five times if you are washing a 1,500-square-foot home. Hand sponges and a sponge mop will help.

After you have washed each wall, wipe the washed areas with rags that have been laundered in baking soda and not in fragrance detergent. This is time-consuming, but it is about as inexpensive as you can get. Available at most markets, baking soda is normally cheap. The end result is a dwelling that will smell and feel fresh for a lengthy period after the treatment.

Let's review the other big indoor problem category: particles.

Particles

Particles include anything that can only be seen under the microscope, such as pollen and mold, plant parts, dust, cat and dog antigen, diesel exhaust, and latex from rubber tires.

Pollen (Please see chapter on Pollen). This is a major player in the world of respiratory problems, and may be an indoor problem in certain cases. We're finding out that it's not just the pollen grain that is allergenic, but the entire plant, which contains many of the same antigens that are present in its pollen.[3] These factors have been understood since at least 1984, with hundreds of documents to provide evidence.

Mold (see Mold section). Indoor mold damage can occur from literally fifty different sources. Wherever there is plumbing, rain, snowfall, or outdoor flooding, there is a potential for water damage and subsequent mold growth within the building. Unlike pollen, the water damage must be dealt with immediately or mold growth will likely result. The damage caused by water may be reimbursable by insurance; usually, the damage caused by mold is not.

Plant parts. Plants give off microscopic particles other than pollen. These particles are also allergenic. Ragweed and juniper are examples. A big part of household dust, plant parts enter the home via tracking on shoes and air currents.

Two things of interest about plant parts: First, as mentioned earlier, they have many of the same antigens as does the pollen from the same plant. Second, they are produced at a different time of year than pollen.

Dust. People aren't allergic or sensitive to dust. They react to the dozens of components that make up dust. These include cat and dog antigen, lead, and pesticides. There are more of these indoors than out-of-doors.

Also in household dust are harmful carbon particles from automotive exhaust and latex from tires. These are not only allergenic unto themselves, but they also aggravate allergies. Solution: keep the home dust-free and remove shoes at the door.

Particle sizes sometimes offer a clue to their origin. For example, most homes with garages have carbon soot in the air of the home. Most soot particles are in the kitchen or areas nearest the garage entry. A wide variety of microscopic soot sizes can be found here. The larger particles settle out as the air circulates through the home, with the very smallest particles in the master bedroom because it is distant from the garage.

Indoor combustion yields fine particles that are extremely dangerous for a number of reasons. Smoking, cooking, and the burning of firewood, or kerosene leads to the formation of soft furnishings like carpeting, cloth armchairs and sofas, porous drapes, and bedspreads. They retain dust. If you have these items, then vacuum them slowly and carefully.

For example, carpets are functional, add visual and physical warmth, and offer protection. Carpet care should follow manufacturers' recommendations. Most people don't. The common practice is to vacuum quickly, with a unit that has poor suction. It's more effective to vacuum slowly and cross-wise, with a cleaner that doesn't leak and contains upgraded bags.

In the case where old carpeting is present in schools or office buildings, it is not uncommon to find an extremely high concentration of carpet fibers in the air and in the settled dust.

Keep the master bedroom as simple as a motel room. Throw the bedspread in the clothes dryer (on the "air" setting) at least once weekly to shake loose the dust, and avoid the use of fragrance products in the washer and dryer. You have to spend hours each night breathing in their fragrance.

Go through the home room by room and decide how to simplify it. Remove or reorganize items that are dust catchers. This is not an idle recommendation. The amount of dust in the home, along with its constituents, can make a significant contribution to better or worse respiratory health for the occupants—adults, children, and pets.

Make sure you dust items above eye level.

Outside, you may want to plant a stand of fast-growing wind-breaking trees. (Oleanders are discouraged, as explained below.) A fence with gaps between the slats is better than a solid fence for purposes of repair.

Oleander (*Nerium oleander*) poses an interesting problem. Originally of Mediterranean origin, the plant can grow to a height of over fifteen feet.

The poisonous properties of the oleander have been known for centuries. Two principle types of poisons are present throughout the entire plant. One of them is a cardiac glycoside, which, when ingested, can cause nausea, vomiting, accelerated or decreased heartbeat, and cardiac arrest. Ingestion of its leaves, stems, and flowers has caused the death of dairy animals and has poisoned many children. Burning the plant can have a similar effect.

Probably more importantly, the plant produces a great deal of leaf debris. This debris can degrade into fine particles, and these are carried on the wind or are stirred up upon raking. The poisons are present in these particles and are weather stable. Under these circumstances, once they are inhaled, their toxicity to humans is unknown. I have long considered that an interesting study would be to compare the amount of oleander debris near homes and the number of particles that can become airborne. Once that is established, subsequent clinical studies might find a correlation between various illnesses of home occupants and the number of airborne oleander particles.

Thus, what is in airborne particles can be hazardous from numerous standpoints, from the allergenic nature of mold, pollen, plant particles, and diesel exhaust carbon, to the poisonous nature of debris from the oleander (and probably other plants), to food and insect particles in household dust, to pesticides that attach to the dust. Fungal toxins associated with mold will be addressed separately in the section on mold.

Chapter 2

Fixing the Dust Problem

While there are three thousand cases of cancer each year due to outdoor pollutants, there are twenty thousand cases due to indoor pollutants.

Dust (and everything in it) found in old carpets, sofas, and mattresses appears to be a major source of toxic exposure to us. They can have four hundred times the level of carcinogens and lead compared with bare floors, windowsills, and other bare surfaces. This is because they have not been maintained or cleaned adequately over the years. Surfaces are another problem, because lead is commonly found in almost all dust samples taken from windowsills and other surfaces. The more dust, the more lead.

So where do we go from here?

Air the home on a regular basis (not in pollen or mold season if you are sensitive to these allergens) or use a well-maintained evaporative cooler, or both. In general, ventilation is a good thing.

Use a quality air filter, such as a pleated filter, in your central air-handling system. This includes a good-quality air purifier for the master bedroom. Hardware stores will carry a variety of air filters. Regular damp dusting of surfaces and regular vacuuming along with regular house care is called for. (See chapter on vacuum cleaners.)

Here are other solutions:

1. Remove your shoes upon entering the home. This will decrease the amount of substances you track indoors — lead, pollen, mold, plant parts, and pesticides — by a factor of as much as ten. Even front and backdoor shoe-wipe mats can make a big difference. This is probably the most important recommendation of all.

2. Use an efficient vacuum cleaner with a power head once a week on rugs and floors (twice a week with a crawling child in the home).

3. Once a month, vacuum and/or wet-wash surfaces that you may touch (furniture, windowsills, children's toys, and car interiors). Hand-vacuum with a power-head on plush upholstery.

4. Choose furniture, floor coverings, and curtains that are easy to clean. Bare floors, flat rugs, and flat upholstery are easier to clean than plush upholstery and porous curtains.

5. Clean carpets annually with a truck-mounted hot water extraction system.

6. Clean air ducts once every few years (Please see chapter on air duct cleaning.)

7. Use the least toxic products available for cleaning and other home uses.

8. Use your bathroom and kitchen exhaust fans.

9. Vacuum area rugs on both sides, as a single pass on one

side will only remove 5 to 15 percent of the dirt. And it is the dirt we are after.

10. Air dry-cleaned clothes outside whenever possible for at least a day before wearing them. Realize, however, that unless they are aired in warm to hot weather, the perchloroethylene will not evaporate.

There are a lot of advantages to organizing the home for reasons of health. One nice thing is that it can be done inexpensively. Ultimately, you will have more free time because cleaning will be easier. While it may not be fun, it provides the excuse to throw away, give away, or store items that you no longer need or want.

Papers lying around, books and videotapes that should be behind cabinet doors, and a mess in general is often part of our lives. It doesn't have to be. Experts agree, if dust and allergies are your problem, do yourself a favor and reorganize your home.

Some of the worst dust-catching areas of the home are as follows:

1. Countertops: Kitchen appliances should be put back in cabinets after they have been cleaned.

2. Areas above eye level: This includes the top of the refrigerator, pictures, window ledges, and ceiling fan blades.

3. Desk and work area: Part of our clutter problem is that we just don't know where to put things. If the philosophy of "When in doubt, throw it out" is too drastic for you, then create more files. The office area is like any other area. It can be a runaway problem.

4. Books and bookcases: Not only the shelves but the tops of the books retain dust. See if you can find some way to enclose those books. Simplify your home and the master bedroom as well.

5. Decorative items: These are the toughest to clean because they have so many grooves and dust-settling areas. They are so personal that we hate to put them into storage. However, pictures on walls retain less dust than do pictures standing up, and items behind glass gather little dust. Locate appropriate cabinets to display your items behind glass.

6. Closets: Nobody ever dusts them, but there are numerous ways to reorganize the clutter in closets so that it's possible. You can purchase closet reorganizers, or you can do your own shelf building and improvising. Throw out the old. Spend time in those closets. Once the closets have been totally reorganized they will be like new additions to the home.

7. Under the beds and underneath the fridge: Anybody who has ever looked in either of these places knows about dust balls or dust bunnies.

Chapter 3

Plants That Clean the Air

As early as 1990, the National Aeronautics and Space Administration (NASA) concluded a series of experiments to determine which plants were most efficient at cleaning the air, according to the journal *Environment*. The results of a two-year joint study with the Associated Landscape Contractors of America have been released. (Online references to this study are readily available.[4,5,6])

NASA's research into clean air directly relates to the future of interplanetary manned spacecraft, space stations, and space colonies, as it is necessary to purify and detoxify the initial oxygen supply due to the impossibility of providing enough oxygen for years of habitation.

This knowledge has more down-to-earth applications as well. Sealed buildings have less exchange of fresh outdoor air for stale indoor air. This permits a buildup of toxic or stale air-related chemicals such as glues, formaldehyde, vapors from cleaning products, and carbon dioxide.

Through experimentation, NASA confirmed what millions already knew: that other gases can be absorbed by many common houseplants to clean the air. But they have gone two steps further by identifying the gases and the plants.

NASA found that combining plant foliage with a bed of activated carbon creates a filtration system with a cleansing capability much greater than that of the plants alone.

Researchers still don't know how many plants it takes to remove a certain amount of pollutants in the home or office. A plant in an experimental test chamber that absorbs a specific amount of benzene under controlled scientific conditions is a lot different than a plant in a bedroom that has variable light, heat, air currents, and exposure to chemicals.

Despite these problems, NASA's estimates say that one Janet Craig dracaena (*Dracaena deremensis*) would purify the air in a room that measures ten feet by fifteen feet with an eight foot ceiling, but others caution about turning your home into a rain forest based on limited information.

Your local botanist and plant shops may be of assistance to you in your pursuit of learning about the relationship between clean indoor air and plants.

Recently, the Associated Landscape Contractors of America established the Foliage for Clean Air Council to publicize the NASA study results. Sixteen plants were found to significantly remove formaldehyde, carbon monoxide, dust, benzene, and trichloroethylene present in buildings.

Formaldehyde is found in hundreds of household products, including clothing, furniture, cleaners, cosmetics, and particle board. It is especially concentrated in mobile homes.

Benzene is found in tobacco smoke, gasoline, synthetic fibers, plastics, detergents, and rubber.

Trichloroethylene is found in dry cleaning, inks, paints, varnishes, lacquers, and adhesives.

The plants that remove these chemicals from the air are listed below:

> » Chinese evergreen (*Aglaonema* "Silver Queen")
> » Spider plant (*Chlorophytum elatum*)
> » Pot mum (*Chrysanthemum x morifolium*)
> » Janet Craig dracaena (*Dracaena deremensis* "Janet Craig")
> » Corn plant (*Dracaena fragrans* "Massangeana")

- » Elephant's ear philodendron (*Philodendron domesticum*)
- » Heart-leaf philodendron (*Philodendron scandens oxycardium*)
- » English ivy (*Hedera helix*)
- » Banana tree (*Musa*)
- » Reed palm (*Chamaedorea seifrizii*)
- » Gerbera daisy (*Gerbera jamesonii*)
- » Golden pothos (*Epipremnum aureum*)
- » Snake plant (*Sansevieria trifasciata* "Laurentii")
- » Peace lily (*Spathiphyllum* "Mauna Loa")

The ability of plants to remove dust was a noteworthy surprise finding; by providing a bed of activated charcoal over the potting soil, the air purification was enhanced.

The applications of this research are obvious: we may use many more indoor plants in mobile and conventional homes and offices to purify the air. The caveat is that we must endeavor to maintain the plants in a healthy condition for maximum effect, and to lessen the amount of mold growth on dead and dying leaves.

Burge and coworkers found that modest numbers of undisturbed houseplants (up to ten per room) contribute minimally to aeroallergen prevalence in homes. However, especially under greenhouse conditions, plantings can harbor abundant fungus growth that may become airborne, especially when agitated directly.[4,7]

Chapter 4

Nontoxic Cleaners

The following is a guide that you may wish to further research due to the presence of ample and readily available materials on the subjects. (Please see the section on safe household cleaning.)

One may reduce daily personal chemical exposures by selecting soaps without artificial color or fragrance. A nontoxic shampoo can be made with one part olive or avocado oil, two parts distilled water, and four parts castile soap. Baking soda and cornstarch in equal amounts create a nontoxic deodorant powder for adults.

Herbs such as onions and mint can be planted around buildings to discourage entry of insects. Boric acid powder is a safer alternative to sprays for ants and roaches. Slugs and snails are easy victims for beer traps. For pets, toxic flea collars can be replaced with herbal collars and ointments made from eucalyptus or rosemary. Brewer's yeast in an animal's diet also discourages fleas and *ticks*. Instead of carcinogenic mothballs, try cedar chips or lavender flowers. A solution of soap and water can be sprayed on the leaves of houseplants to kill pests.[8,9,10]

An all-purpose cleaner can be made by combining a teaspoon each of liquid soap and borax in a quart of warm water and adding a squeeze of lemon.

Half a cup of borax to a gallon of water makes a household disinfectant.

Linoleum floors are effectively cleaned with half a cup of white vinegar to a gallon of water.

Baking soda substitutes for scouring powder and removes porcelain stains.

Wine and coffee cup stains can be removed with moist salt.

Carpet upholstery stains may be removed with club soda.

Rust spots on clothing can be bleached out with lemon juice and sunlight.

Spills in the oven should be sprinkled with salt immediately, then moistened and brushed with baking soda after the oven cools.

We have been led to believe that hazardous commercial products are best for carrying out household chores. Certainly, in their own way, they do the job. But our use of these products is only a conditioned habit that can be broken. Take a look at an inexpensive product that will not only lighten the load on your respiratory tract, but will also save money and not take up much space under your sink: the lemon. (See Section 13, Chapter 1 on the many uses for the lemon.)

Chapter 5

Home Storage of Cleaning Agents

"Solvent" is a very broad term encompassing a wide range of liquids that are capable of dissolving or dispersing other substances. They are found in many products commonly used at home and at work. For example, solvents include paints, varnishes, adhesives, pesticides, and cleaning solutions, and are among the chemicals most frequently implicated by chemically sensitive (CS) patients. The volatile organic compounds associated with sick building syndrome are in large part solvent vapors.

There is a curious range of effects caused by solvents on normal people, according to Ashford and Miller (see Selected References), such as being alert, enthusiastic, energetic, and witty, or becoming tense, jittery, and argumentative. There is also a withdrawal phase whereby normal people report allergy-like symptoms, and CS people report fatigue, depression, headache, and joint aches.

If you are seeking escape from solvent vapors, be aware that there must be plenty of ventilation to dilute the chemical gas. This means getting a lot of fresh air during and after painting (as well as seeking a paint that uses a water base, and taking plenty of rest breaks).

In the average home, a fair number of solvents, paints, varnishes, detergents, household cleaning products, aerosols, and similar products are stored under the sinks, in laundry room cabinets, on garage shelves, and in other locations. It may seem obvious, but we don't always close containers properly. Wash or wipe spills that may have occurred on the side of the container or on the shelf, and properly dispose of the rag. Don't just throw it in the trash without containing it in a plastic trash bag.

Also, obtain a plastic container of appropriate size to store these substances. Obtain a tight-fitting top for it. If you are going to go this route, then wipe down the shelves first to remove the odor of chemicals that has layered onto them. Use a damp washcloth and baking soda, or a dilute solution of trisodium phosphate (TSP).

Chapter 6

Newsprint Breakthrough

Over the past several years (if not decades), there have been a number of rumors, personal reports, word-of-mouth testimonies, and medical cautions regarding the potential hazards of newsprint ink. It seems as if everybody has an opinion on this subject. Reportedly, there is a cause-and-effect relationship between this ink and symptoms in people sensitive to volatile organic compounds (VOCs), but it has been difficult to prove. Even sensitivity to VOCs in general, to the extent that clinical symptoms may be long-lasting, is met by skepticism by much of the medical community.

The matter brings forth the following questions: just exactly what is in newsprint, and where is the industry headed?

Historically, inks were comprised of chrome, lead, and flammable solvents. Paper dust was as much a problem to the newspaper recipient as it was to the newspaper worker.

In 1989, President Bush proposed legislation to update and strengthen the Clean Air Act, which was passed in 1970. A major portion of that bill is directed toward decreasing VOCs that are found in hydrocarbon-based petroleum inks.

In this regard, for several years research has been ongoing with the hopes of completely switching to soybean-based inks (SI). It has been found that SIs have several advantages over petroleum-based (PI) inks: SIs do not emit VOCs at nearly the rate of PIs. They are environmentally safer in that they are biodegradable.[12] There is less ink transfer to the hands (especially when no-rub inks become universally adapted). Soybeans are grown in the United States, in the Midwest. The price is comparable to PI when colored ink is used. Importantly, much of the ink is recycled.[11]

Most newspaper inks use the same soy oil that is used in cooking. Add to it a small amount of coloring agents and binder (resins), and there you have a price that is competitive with PI. At the end of the first marketing year, according to the American Soybean Association, six newspapers were using SI. One thousand newspapers were using the ink at the end of the second year. After three years of availability, soy ink was being used by one-quarter to one-third of the nation's 9,100 newspapers, including half of the daily 1,500 newspapers.[12] A number of Midwestern states have passed laws mandating the use of SI for state government printing.

When newspapers convert from PI to SI, it is due to a number of factors: environmental safety, availability, less exposure to VOCs by staff and the public, better recyclability of newsprint, better color, and pricing competitive with PI. This latter is important, as a newspaper with a daily circulation of seventy-five thousand spends more than $700,000 yearly for newsprint ink.

Admittedly, there is a catch. As noted by virtually all parties involved, SI works best for colored newsprint, advertising fliers, brochures, catalogues, and similar products. The drawback comes when black ink is involved. The reason is cost. Surprisingly, it costs almost twice as much to print in black as it does to print in color per unit. This is because of the difference in price between soy oil (the ink solvent) and petroleum oil, and the differences in cost between the inks used for each.

According to the American Soybean Association, about one hundred million bushels of soybeans are used per year to manufacture a wide variety of ink; thirty million of these are used for soy-based newspaper solvent. Use of soy oil is a function of supply and demand, and as more soy is used for oil purposes, the cost will come down.

The rub comes here: Because the Department of Agriculture limits the amount of soy that is grown in the United States, the price of soy stays high compared to open market economy prices. This forces the print media to stay with petroleum-based oils.

In summary, new no-rub inks and new petroleum oils that have a low content of petroleum-based volatile organic compounds, lacking in carcinogens, help the industry to maintain a quality black ink for printing. When the price of soy oil becomes competitive with the price of petroleum oil, then the industry will switch to soy oil, which has virtually no VOCs.[13]

Chapter 7

Create a Clean Room

Soft furnishings and dust go together. So do under-bed and under-refrigerator areas.

The master bedroom may be the worst of the indoor worlds in terms of both the airborne and settled dust and the volatile organic compounds (VOCs) that originate in the bathroom. Add to this the length of time we are exposed to the particles and VOCS, combine that with our own sensitivities, and we have a bad mixture. Our goal is to control the level of dust in the home, especially in the bedroom, where we spend so much time.

(As an aside, pole lamps and other light fixtures capture insects, which burn when the light is on. Keep these areas clean.)

There should be a certain pleasure in knowing that there is at least one area of the home that is allergen free—a clean room.

When we can create a clean room, then our reaction to the environment in general will improve. Have some fun and re-organize.

The clean room needs to be as simple and plain as possible, with a minimum of soft furnishings such as armchairs, lace curtains, carpeting, and porous bedspreads. Furniture should be simple, not ornate. In general, the less furniture in the room, the better it is for your respiratory health.

Use simple bedspreads that you can throw in the clothes dryer; then you can run the dryer on "air" to remove the dust.

Dacron, *polyester*, or other synthetic fibers can be used for pad fillings as well as for pillows. Never use feather, kapok, foam rubber, or cotton pillows, as these can break down in time and either leak particles into the air or become contaminated with microbes that obtain their moisture from sweaty heads.

Use washable plain cotton curtains in the room. Avoid drapes that require dry cleaning, as the commercial dry cleaning fluids outgas over a long period of time. Avoid any shag or soft velvety fabric for curtains. Do not use venetian blinds unless they are vertical. Keep it simple.

No shoes allowed in the bedroom. If you have an air purifier, keep it running at night. You will soon get accustomed to the background noise, which will override other sounds of the night.

Weather-strip the windows to minimize the influx of dust.

Clean out the closet and keep only the most frequently worn clothes in it. Clothes retain dust, and they also emit odors from fragrance detergent, fabric softeners, and chemicals, such as formaldehyde, added to new clothing. The idea is to minimize your exposure to airborne irritants, whether they are particles or gases. This means that you will have to find space somewhere else in the home to put the clothing you do not wear quite so often. Winter clothes should be bagged during the warmer months. Vacuum packing works well to minimize space. Do not permit clothing or papers to lie carelessly about.

Most people pick the master bedroom for their clean room. Keep this room as simple as possible. Make a game out of changing your lifestyle a little bit. After all, it is a free way to reduce your health risk.

Wall hangings should be minimized because dust will settle on the top surface above eye level.

Discourage the use of bookcases for the same reason, and

minimize the use of ornaments and small items that generate more dust than pleasure.

Do not use insecticide sprays or powders in the bedroom. Many of them contain allergens or chemical irritants. Avoid the use of deodorizers and mothballs. The vast majority of them have been found to be carcinogenic.

Blankets and clothing stored for several months should be thoroughly aired out-of-doors or tumbled in the clothes dryer before use.

Remember that the master bedroom is usually connected to the master bath, and the master bathroom can be a real trouble spot unless it is well maintained. This is because it contains numerous fragrance products such as toilet paper, facial tissue, soaps, cosmetics, lotions, hairsprays, shampoos, body talc, conditioners, perfumes, and deodorants. Also present are various cleaning agents, polishes, and solvents. The odors from all of these communicate directly into the master bedroom and, of course, you get the full dose while in the bathroom.

What to do here? Keep just the bare minimum of supplies in the master bathroom and move the rest somewhere else. Scrub out the storage shelves with a solution of baking soda (one-half cup to a bucket of warm water) to absorb the leftover odors. And use the fan frequently. That is what it's for.

There is mounting evidence that houseplants are beneficial in terms of removing odors and dust from home air. However, most of the reports recommend against plants in the home environment of a patient who is dust sensitive because dust gathers on their leaves. Others say that that is the whole point. If you must have plants in the bedroom, the state of health of the plants is probably more important than any other factor, this is because diseased plants liberate more mold spores into the air than healthy plants.

Keep the bedroom dust free with frequent cleaning. Wipe exposed floors, shelves, tables, and other furniture with a damp cloth oiled with a mixture of one part lemon juice and one or two parts cooking oil or olive oil.

Assuming your ducts are not leaking, you should now have a dust-free and smell-free room. So no matter what else is going on outside as far as wind, pollen, mold, or irritants, this room will be a safe haven for you.

These are all proven methods for exposure reduction. They are not extreme, and allergists and researchers around the world recommend them. Creating a safe room is important as it is something we can all do without spending a lot of money.

Chapter 8

Respiratory Problems and Indoor Heat

What would you say if the weatherman forecasted moderate to cool temperatures over the next several days, weeks, or even months with the relative humidity at or below 20 percent? Should you be concerned?

Second, do you have a particular ailment that is going around? The symptoms are dry and scratchy throat, sometimes to the point of soreness in the morning, and itching eyes, scalp, and skin. Do you talk like a frog when you wake up?

Are your allergies activated both outdoors and indoors even though the usual allergens are at a low level outside and you can't think of any way that your indoor lifestyle has changed?

Finally, are you still having problems even if you don't have allergies? Welcome to the world of winter with the heater turned on.

Depending on the amount of draft and leakage in your home, the level of indoor humidity will vary, but expect the vast majority of homes, apartments, and other buildings to experience a sharp decrease during the cool evening hours. Space heaters create the fewest issues; central forced air creates the most. The higher the heat and the tighter the home, the worse the problem becomes.

Some scientists believe that dry air is a major factor in aggravating underlying respiratory disorders. They believe that the respiratory tract becomes primed when exposed to a low level of moisture for a period of time. This fits right in with what is known about asthma.

So, we go home (or to school or to work), turn on the heating supply, and burn off the moisture. If it's at home, then it may be all night. Senior citizens and shut-ins could be exposed to extremely dry conditions for lengthy periods of time. In the world of indoor air quality, this is called being out of the comfort zone.

Why are people reacting as if it is pollen season already? Because you don't necessarily have to be exposed to a high dose of new allergens to have symptoms under dry conditions; the same old ones will do just fine.

What to do? Be aware that you are not catching some dreaded disease. A glass of water next to the night stand and periodic sips during the night should help the throat and add needed moisture to a dehydrated respiratory tract.

Hairspray dries the skin; moisturizer helps retain the moisture. Also, to add moisture to the air, do not operate your cooking range or bathroom fans while cooking or showering.

One thing that is common to virtually all homes: a central heat supply. Thought needs to be given prior to turning on that central heat source

Let's take a close look at why the central heater frequently stinks when it is first turned on for the season, and why it causes so much respiratory distress.

There are a number of reasons. First, the heater unit, like any other area of the home, accumulates dust and worn fibers. The difference is that this area doesn't get dusted. The fibers come from natural and synthetic materials in carpets, furniture, draperies, and clothing. They include natural fibers, such as cotton and wool. They include synthetics such as nylon, rayon, and polyester.

The gases that are released are the same as or similar to those released during a fire. When these fibers are heated or burned, they give off small amounts of annoying, if not toxic, gases. These gases may include *hydrogen cyanide* and acrolein.[14,15] Both of these byproducts of combustion can cause headaches and nausea, among other symptoms.

Hydrogen cyanide is poisonous, and it is a respiratory and eye irritant. It is generated during the burning of grass clippings, weeds, cotton, paper products, silk, and man made products including plastics, nylon, and soft furnishings. This includes their fibers.

Acrolein is also a constituent of cigarette smoke. It is released when fats, wood, some plant particles, and certain foods are burned, and is produced readily during cooking fires or by burned grease that settles on the heating unit. It is a highly toxic respiratory irritant that causes tearing, affects the mucous membranes, and causes skin irritation. It reacts readily with other chemicals. Acrolein was actually used as a chemical weapon during World War I until it was banned.

Also, aerosols that we use during the year will find their way to the heating unit and the duct system to become warmed, heated, and sent back into the home. These aerosols may include pesticides, herbicides, furniture polishes, and cleaning solvents.

In addition, there can be a certain amount of condensate in the ducts and furnace where microorganisms may flourish. They can get burned off, too. And remember that basic smells of any home are a lot more noticeable when they are warmed.

Gas furnaces have an additional problem in that there is a distinctive odorant, *mercaptan*, in the gas. This is added so that you will not confuse it with another smell in the event of a gas leak. Uneven heat at the first startup leads to uneven burning, and the odorant is a lot more noticeable than at subsequent startups.

Many persons become ill at the smell of first heat because of the low concentration of gases and particles that are being burned off. Some do not use the heater for the remainder of the winter, thinking that the smell is permanent. Be kind to yourself. Ventilate. It may be cold outside, but open the windows a little, then turn on the heat. It shouldn't take long for the odors and the VOCs to dissipate. Chances are you will now have a warm home that has little or no smell for the rest of the season.

On a final note, if you have had a gas furnace for a number of years, then you need to be aware that there may be hairline cracks in the heat exchanger, which means that deadly carbon monoxide gas could be entering your home. Call your local gas company or a licensed contractor to check out the furnace for leaks.

Chapter 9
Smells from New Carpeting

What causes the smell in new carpeting?

The backing on a carpet is rubberized, and a chemical known as 4-phenylcyclohexene (4-PC) used in the backing can be smelled at very low levels. Synthetic carpets will have more odor than natural-fiber carpets. This may come as a surprise to many readers, but it has been many years since formaldehyde was used in domestic carpets.

A carpet consists of face yarns attached to primary backing. This is usually coated with latex rubber to lock the yarn to the backing. Sometimes, a secondary backing is added for stability. The rubber is a *styrene*-butadiene complex that produces some volatile organic compound (VOC) emissions. The best known is 4-PC. Its odor is detectable at an extremely low concentration, and this is the odor that most people associate with new carpeting. Other emissions include styrene, decane, toluene, xylene, and a variety of other hydrocarbons.

Commercial carpeting used in offices and schools is typically glued down to a concrete surface that has been prepared with a sealer or adhesive.

Carpet adhesive is a mixture of synthetic rubber, resins, and fillers. When solvents are used to dissolve the resins into a liquid, more than 90 percent of its VOCs are produced.[16] Because of this problem, adhesive manufacturers are developing low-solvent and solvent-free adhesives and seam sealers.

The glues used with commercial carpeting emit most of the VOCs—not the carpet itself.[17] Still, the latex backing in household carpets releases a significant level of VOCs into that environment, although not nearly as much as do the painted walls in a new home. Certain individuals are more reactive to these odors than are others. (An odor is not considered a health effect.)

After carpet installation, the building ventilation system should be run at maximum air and normal temperature for seventy-two hours. The home, business, or school should be opened as much as possible during this three-day period. Exhaust fans can be placed in strategic locations.

Be aware that ceiling tiles, duct liners, and soft furnishings are capable of absorbing VOCs and outgassing those same VOCs.

For home use, fresh air ventilation will, in almost all cases, remove carpet VOCs within a two-to-three-day period. In some cases, activated charcoal filters in a polyester matrix are available for the central air supply and return air ducts. These can be used in circumstances where air dilution is not tenable. Activated charcoal is inexpensive and absorbs many of the VOCs emitted from new carpeting (i.e., carpet and pad), but be aware that it has a limited life span. Eventually the carbon will become saturated and may require several filter changes.

In all circumstances, new carpeting should be vacuumed in a slow cross-wise manner to remove residual fibers.

Old carpeting should be thoroughly vacuumed prior to removal. Afterward, the floor should be damp-mopped. This will minimize the amount of dust generated during carpet removal and installation.

In schools or offices, heavy traffic areas should be vacuumed daily while light or medium traffic areas can be vacuumed once or twice weekly.

The home carpet that is merely tacked down has very little

in the way of VOC emissions, although glue is occasionally used to attach the pad to the slab.

The Carpet and Rug Institute (CRI), which represents the vast majority of carpet manufacturers, tests batches of carpet on a regular basis. In the past the Consumer Product Safety Commission has requested more frequent testing, as batches of carpet vary considerably in their chemical composition. When the carpet meets CRI standards, it is issued an indoor air quality label. Be aware that this is not a label of safety for the consumer.

A number of years ago, the Environmental Protection Agency laid twenty thousand square feet of new carpeting in its eastern headquarters and hundreds of workers complained or became ill.

Neither the CRI nor EPA links emissions from carpets with specific health effects. The key word here is "specific," as individuals can react differently to the same volatile organic compounds. The most frequent effects of low-level exposures to VOCs are stimulation of the senses, inflammation of exposed tissues, including eye and throat irritation, and stress reactions, such as headache and fatigue.[18]

Chapter 10

Low-Emission Paint

Paints of today are much higher quality than those of a couple of decades ago. At that time they contained lead and a high level of what was known as white spirit, or Stoddard solvent. *These are paraffin*-derived solvents used in degreasing and cleaning, lacquers, varnishes, preservatives, and asphalt products.

The water-base paints of today can include water, acrylic latex paint, latex primer and enamel, biocides, surfactants, white pigments and extender pigments, latex monomer precursors, solvents and *cosolvents*, *driers*, *plasticizers*, *amines*, and various volatile substances. Some of these have a pungent odor.

Though an improvement, water-base paints can irritate the skin and mucous membranes. The volatile substances include ammonia, *butyl acrylate*, *styrene*, *white spirit*, and formaldehyde.

Painters should always maintain good ventilation when painting, and preferably when they are finished painting as well. Office workers and family members should not have to endure the hazards of breathing chemicals released from paints in a confined space.

While drying, oil-base paints emit a very high level of irritating and toxic VOCs—much more than wall coverings, wood products, and carpets combined. Paints are a major contributor to the irritating smell of a new home, much more so than carpeting. Often, they contribute to a great deal of respiratory illness, headaches, nausea, dizziness, and other symptoms in the average residence. If a newly painted home is closed up during hot, humid weather, then the smell absorbs into the walls and carpets (and furnishings) and will outgas for weeks or months.

The VOCs found in many paints include such toxics as xylene, styrene, benzene, and decane. Read the material safety data sheet available online or at the paint store for more information.

One problem with low-emission paints is that they lack good opacity; therefore they are thinner. The white spirits have been removed, along with lead, benzene, xylene, and thickeners. As a result, they are similar to whitewash and can't cover scratches or old paint very well. Plan on using a couple of coats of this type of paint.

Many paint manufacturers now make low-emission paints, and many other companies are coming into the fold. Ask any paint dealer if they carry the right product and ask to see the material safety data sheet. There may be some dealers who sell these paints in your area.

Chapter 11

The Office Environment

Some of the health issues in today's offices include lack of fresh air, cigarette smoke from the clothing of workers, paints, carpeting, cleaners, perfumes, formaldehyde, pesticides, ozone, and plastics from electronic equipment.[18] Also, carbon particles from diesel exhaust may be present as a result of leaky air filters, and control of dust may be poorly managed. Your own experiences may allow you to add some items to this list.

Carbonless copy paper is made with microencapsulated color formers on the back and color formers on the front of the paper sheets. When pressure is applied by a ballpoint pen, the dyes in the capsules are dissolved in various oils and other chemicals. These include *phenyls*, hydrocarbons, *ethane*, naphthalene, chlorinated paraffins (waxes), and benzene-containing chemicals.[19]

The developers most commonly used in the United States are phenolic resins—that is, hardeners related to benzene.

NIOSH reports that there have been no conclusive studies linking health effects in the office with this paper. However, its use in poorly ventilated offices should be discontinued on general principle.[20] Finally, if you have to go outside the building to smoke, be aware that sometimes the fresh air intake is just over your head outside the front door.

One of the most common problems in the office environment is the copy room. This room usually consists of numerous machines in a confined space. It is common for several people to use the machines at a time, and ventilation in the area is poor. Ventilation here is the key to fresher air. Fresh air dilutes the machine byproducts that can irritate many people. Ozone is one example of such an irritant in this setting. It is produced by any electrically operated device, can combine with other chemicals in the air to create free radicals, and can be a respiratory irritant.

Mimeograph fluid is another irritant that is still used in lower-budget offices and schools, as mimeographing is more economical than photocopying. The mimeograph process is over one hundred years old and utilizes an organic solvent (methyl alcohol) that is used in some dry-cleaning processes, the VOCs of which are readily dissipated into the air.

Another problem in the office is an extremely high level of airborne and settled dust. The dust often contains a very high concentration of carbon particles from vehicular exhaust and a very high concentration of worn carpet fibers that can number in the thousands per cubic meter. In addition, because numerous people are usually present in the typical office, there is a significant amount of tracking of dirt indoors on shoes. This is ground to a fine powder that either settles into the carpeting or becomes airborne. The areas of the highest concentration of settled dust are the ones most trafficked, such as outside elevators, the conference room, and main walkways. An occasional careful deep steam cleaning by professionals will help to remove a great deal of the settled dust. Anything less than that is only partial dust management, which will have a brief effect on the dust in the carpeting, and hence that which becomes airborne. Be aware that you may want to decline the use of a carpet degreaser during its cleaning for a couple of reasons. First, fragrance is frequently added to degreasers and will pose a respiratory hazard to workers. Second, they cost more. Grease stains can be removed by the regular cleaning staff as a point of interest. Preferably, the deep steam cleaning should be accomplished after Friday's workday is finished, on Saturday, or prior to a holiday to provide ample time for the carpet to dry completely prior to beginning of the next workday. Why a dry carpet? Shoe tracks are unsightly.

Again, dusting above eye level should be part of a cleaning crew's chores.

A conscientious cleaning staff and a good-quality vacuum cleaner will help reduce the indoor particle load. This should be coupled with a balanced airflow, which hopefully can be arranged with building management, and an upgraded return register air filter, or one that is centrally located and can be changed on a regular basis.

Balancing the airflow will provide more air to the portions of the facility that get the most traffic. This helps dilute contaminants and provide an influx of new air.

Finally, check the cleaning supplies. Ensure that they are as odor-free as possible and are EPA approved.

Please also refer to the chapter on mold in the office for more information.

Chapter 12

Arts and Crafts

Question: What business sells acetone, methyl ethyl ketone, toluene, xylene, derivatives of trichloroethane, hexane isomers, aliphatic hydrocarbons, propane, diacetone alcohol, turpentine, linseed oil, d-limonene, wood stain, spray enamel, epoxy paint, and adhesive caulk?

Answer: Art supply stores. These stores sell graphic and art supplies to amateur and professional painters, architects, schools and parks, and recreational art students.

Historically, artists, like painters, have encountered toxic heavy metals such as cadmium, iron, lead, silver, and gold; toxic aerosols; and in more recent times, VOCs made from petroleum products. Nowadays, most art supply stores are environmentally attuned, and like many other related businesses, are becoming health conscious.

Exposure to hazardous substances in art supplies occurs by three routes: inhalation, ingestion, and skin absorption.[20] Hand-to-mouth contact cannot be ruled out for anyone. Those exposed to potentially toxic materials in craft materials should be aware that many solvents can be absorbed through the skin and enter the bloodstream, thus affecting various organ systems, including the liver, kidneys, and central nervous system.

For millennia, the arts and crafts business/industry was loaded with poisonous materials. These ranged from heavy metals such as lead, gold, silver, and cadmium. They were found in dyes, stains, oils, and solvents that were inhaled, or entered the body via absorption through the skin.[20] In recent years the industry has responded to social pressure and common sense, and it has gone to great lengths to create nontoxic water-base materials. The xylene-free nontoxic marker is but one of many examples.

More solvents are moving away from a petroleum-base toward more water-base types. These include water-base acrylics. One important example is markers. The chemicals previously used could dissolve neurological tissue; this became a real problem with teachers and with children, who were more susceptible to all manner of VOCs (and heavy metals). Today, many markers are labeled as nontoxic and do not give off VOCs.

Pigments used for watercolors and oil painting contain fewer heavy metals with each passing year, just as home paints have eliminated lead and are generally safer than the paints of past decades.

Another example is canned air used for airbrushing. Most propellants are now environmentally safe, with isobutane as one of the most common types.

As always, fresh air ventilation, cannot be overemphasized when one is engaged in the practice of painting.

This discussion also applies to home workshops, summer programs, artists, housepainters and a variety of hobbyists.

The instructor must be aware of the potential problems in order to pass on this information to students. Complacency results when people are unaware of the toxicity related to familiar items.

For example, the deliberate and purposeful smelling of xylene in markers can become psychologically, if not physically habit-forming, as the user attempts to get "high." The practice should be considered very dangerous to brain and lung function by any and all accounts. It's in the same league as glue sniffing because xylene is present in many types of glue. Constant exposure to xylene from markers, even at low doses, can be hazardous over time. This is because xylene and related chemicals such as toluene and benzene are nonpolar solvents. As such, they are soluble in nonpolar tissue like fatty tissue and nervous tissue, which includes the myelin covering over the central nervous system. Overexposure to solvents produces symptoms of sneezing, itching and watery eyes, runny nose, blocked sinuses, coughing spells, headaches, itching and redness of skin, shortness of breath, dizziness, memory loss, fatigue, and neurological disorders.[21]

The next biggest problem, after lack of awareness, is poor ventilation of the work areas. Typically, windows are closed to maintain air-conditioning, or the weather outside does not permit open windows. (As room temperature increases, so does volatilization of solvents and the concomitant increase of their absorption through the skin and mouth.) In addition, entrance doors are often closed to maintain privacy.

There is no readily available and inexpensive type of ventilation that will accommodate the two major potential hazards: solvent vapors and dust created during hobby work.

Ceiling exhaust fans, open windows, and evaporative cooling help remove the vapors, fumes, and particles; these can be very helpful if they are close to the source. But if you have respiratory problems or just want to maintain your hobby in the field of art as safely as possible, then ask your art supplier about safe alternatives to the paints, pigments, and sprays.

Most of the exposure to solvent vapors comes through respiratory intake. Secondarily, the vapors are absorbed by the skin.

Solvent spills are a related problem. They are not uncommon in the classroom or at home. Let's take paint thinner, carbon tetrachloride, as an example here. NIOSH describes this solvent as a colorless liquid with an etherlike odor and tells us that overexposure can lead to central nervous system depression, nausea, vomiting, liver and kidney damage, and cancer.[22]

There is a correct way and an incorrect way to clean up spills. Lack of training in spill mopping and proper disposal of contaminated materials leads to further evaporation of the spilled solvent from the table or floor. As the spill is mopped, the wet paper or cloth frequently comes into contact with the hands. The solvent is absorbed into the skin, blood, muscles, and nerves. Thus, absorbent materials should be used for spill mopping and held with nonabsorbent gloves to minimize chances that there will be contact of the solvent with the hands.[23] Closed foot-operated cans with plastic liners are preferable to open trash cans to contain the vapors for disposal purposes; however, they pose a potential problem for the buildup of explosive gases, unless containers such as those made from Nalgene are utilized.

Small particles generated through carpentry are another potential hazard in arts and crafts classes as well as at home. Wood dust, metallic dust, and clay particles generated through wood and pottery work can reach very high levels indoors where the hobbyist has not created an escape route for the particles. Grinding, sanding, sawing, and similar activities require a dust mask to be worn, a habit which is not widely practiced. Frequently, ear protection is not worn either.

Similar to the Richter Scale as a measurement of intensity of earthquakes, the decibel or dB is a logarithmic scale that is commonly used in the measurement of sound intensity. Let's take a brief look at *decibel* (dB) limits to get an idea of what sound intensities are found in our daily lives.[23,24] (Since this is not a linear scale, 40 is ten times louder than thirty, and 60 is 100 times the level of 40.)

Event	dB (approx.)
Quiet library	30
Refrigerator humming	40
Normal conversation	60
Telephone dial tone	80
Subway train at 200 ft.	95
Motorcycle	95
Automobiles	90
Power tools	105
Rock concert	115
Gun blast	140

At the 90–95 dB level, sustained exposure may lead to hearing loss.

Finally, we must address the issue of overall neatness. This includes the proper storage and labeling of arts and crafts materials such as solvents, cleaners, and finishes. Doing so will go a long way toward reducing the level of vapors in storage lockers and our exposure to them when they are first opened. It will reduce the level of spillages as well as unnecessary skin contact with solvents.

Chapter 13

Choosing a Pest Control Company

At the outset, those who have their indoor environment sprayed monthly and believe that they are chemically sensitive should consider ceasing and desisting. There are many non-toxic methods to control pests and a number of quality and detailed guides available to assist the consumer with ways to rid the home and prevent the habitation of the home by virtually any insect pest.

Certainly, termites, roaches, mites, fleas, *crickets*, and ants need to be controlled, and occasionally, despite our best efforts, we can't eliminate the pests by ourselves. The EPA publishes a guide entitled *Citizen's Guide to Pest Control and Pesticide Safety*.[31] This booklet does not tell us about pesticides per se, but it does tell us about how to choose a pest control company.

There are many reputable pest control companies. If you've decided that you need one to aid you, here are some questions you can ask, according to the booklet.

1. Does the company have a good track record? Don't rely on the company salesman to answer the question; research the answer yourself. Ask your friends and neighbors and check with the local consumer office to see if there have been any complaints. One client related to me that her doctor (a nationally recognized asthma specialist) told her not to have her home sprayed. The doctor's rationale: the recommended sprays contained pyrethrum (related to ragweed) and volatile organic

compounds. The salesperson told her that the doctor did not know what he was talking about; this spray was harmless. While such an experience is a rare one, it points to the fact that you should ask questions of the company and of your doctor.

2. Can the salesman prove that the company is insured? Contractor's general liability insurance, including insurance for sudden and accidental pollution, gives you, as a homeowner, a certain degree of protection should an accident occur while pesticides are being applied in your home. Contractor's workmen's compensation can also protect you, should an employee of the contractor be injured in your home.

3. Is the company licensed? If it is licensed, then there is a certified pesticide applicator present in their office to supervise the work. Make sure the license is current.

4. Does the company stand behind its work, and can you stand behind your part of the bargain? In the case of termite control, a guarantee may be invalidated if structural alterations are made without prior notice to the pest control company.

5. This is most important: is the company willing to discuss the treatment proposed for your home (and the safety of their product), including special instructions you should follow to reduce your exposure to the pesticide?

Most pest control companies are licensed and reputable.

However, the chemicals they use are toxic to life. Frequently, the consumer is not completely informed or does not ask enough questions. You may be consuming more than you know. If there are other methods for pest control, don't be afraid to say no. And check the alternatives. Most, if not all reputable companies will have more than one pesticide on hand and will have a good working knowledge about less toxic agents. Find out about water-base versus oil-base pesticides, the length of time they will last, and the specific cost of the pesticide you are buying. Finally, ask to see the material safety data sheet on each one and compare them.

Chapter 14

The Holiday Season

The holiday season has the potential for all the elements of life's happiness: giving and receiving, friendship, sharing, song and merriment, get-togethers, and lots of food. However, it is also a time when many people become depressed or ill for days or weeks. We tend to blame these problems on financial pressures, a variety of frustrations, and other reasons that are mentally oriented. But consider the depression and illness rate from a physical standpoint—respiratory toxicity and overdosing.

Overdosing the respiratory tract with airborne chemical substances can lead to depression, behavioral changes, and mood swings, and can affect the nervous and muscular systems. Entire scientific journals are devoted to this subject. During the holidays, our exposure to these chemicals occurs over a short intense period of time, as opposed to our continual exposure at a lower dose throughout most of the rest of the year. Some scientists believe that this high-dose exposure tends to make us more sensitive to indoor airborne allergens and food allergens.

Common problem areas

Fireplaces are known trouble spots because of the outdoor and indoor pollution they create. Many woods contain resins and oils, and synthetic logs contain waxes and aldehydes which, when burned, cause significant respiratory and systemic problems from the standpoint of particles and gases released into the air.

Pine trees are not reputed to have an allergenic pollen, but the smell of pine affects a large percentage of the population due to the smell of pinene. Pinene is a terpene, a known respiratory irritant related to turpentine, a paint thinner.

Cleaners and aerosols are widely used to clean the homes during the holiday season. Many of these are pine scented. Most allergists will tell you that this scent affects more people than does the pollen from the pine tree itself.

Fragrances in department stores include those sold and those sprayed onto customers; extra time shopping puts us in closer contact with fragrances in the marketplace and in the homes of others.

Pets consider themselves part of the family and a change in the daily routine is noticeable to them. Depending on the type of pet and the breed, we can expect the animals to be nervous, insecure, and expect them to make more trips outdoors and back indoors. Increased activity on the part of household pets permits extra shedding of allergenic hair, feathers, dander, saliva, and skin oils.

Increased traffic congestion is the rule of thumb.

Colder weather and tighter homes magnify the effects. (Please read the chapter Weather and Your Health.)

There is increased contact with the homes of friends and relatives where there are non-fragrance gases from plastics, indoor heating systems, buildup of carbon dioxide and off-gassing from furnishings and newer construction materials. Cigarette, cigar, and pipe smoke can be figured in there somewhere.

Allow yourself time to get occasional periods of solitude and fresh air during the holiday season. This practice could help a lot in terms of preventing or reducing symptoms.

Some common notes from allergists for the holiday season include the following:

Holiday decorations may cause lung and bronchial irritation, as they can be dusty or moldy when they come out of storage after a year. There may be respiratory symptoms if the family sprays with evergreen or pine scent, or uses incense or perfumed candles. Foods avoided all year because of allergy should not be consumed during the holiday either, and allergenic foods can be disguised. Chief among those foods are wheat gluten, nuts, shellfish, corn, and prepared dishes that contain tomato and cheese.

A well-timed visit to the doctor may provide advice and medication ensuring that the entire season is not spent in bed or in discomfort.

There are a number of reasons why it's tough to make it through the several weeks of the holiday season. It is not only a challenge to our lungs, but to our vitality in general. There are a lot of things that can go wrong, and it doesn't have to be this way if we stay in control. What we are looking at is a combination effect of stress, under-sleeping, and overeating. Granted, this is not too different from the rest of the year for most of us, but the stress and exposure levels are high for an intense period during the holidays. The level of outdoor pollen and mold may be low, but just about any indoor environment has potentially hazardous conditions.

Anybody with respiratory problems is just going to have to take it slow as a matter of habit. What this will do is reduce your sensitivity to indoor dust, fragrances, cleaners, chemicals, smoke, cooking odors, and any gas or particle that goes into the nose or mouth. Stressors, and their attendant negative attitudes, enhance a person's sensitivity to these agents manyfold.

Relax prior to cleaning house. Put on some easy music. Unfortunately, opening the windows with snow and sleet outside won't work, but cracking a few of them just a little for draft purposes just might. Turing on the stovetop and bathroom fans will help exhaust the airborne contaminants that are liberated while the cleaning process is going on. Now you can vacuum and clean slowly to reduce the level of irritants.

Operating the heater or air conditioner is not the same as ventilating a home. It is probably true that most houses have enough leaks in their ductwork to permit the escape of some bad air and the entry of some outdoor air, and this does tend to slightly dilute chemicals or odors within the home. For the most part, however, it does not ventilate a home enough to significantly reduce clinical symptoms. It merely recirculates the same air throughout the house. In the winter we can't do much about it. That's why choosing the right cleaning products is so important. Otherwise, the odors from cleaners and polishes build up, and so does the challenge to better breathing. This adds to the stress and the cycle continues.

Check the filter to your central air-handling system before beginning work to ensure that it is relatively new, or at least not overloaded.

Chapter 15
Holiday Odors

During the holiday season, people feel compelled to look good on a frequent basis. If you have respiratory problems, then you already know that a cosmetology salon is not a place for you. This is especially true this time of year, when they are crowded and the chemical overload in the air is likely to be extremely high.

Cut back on perfumes, colognes, fragrances, and after-shaves. This practice will ensure that we offend fewer people who come to visit us or who invite us to visit them.

There are scores of reports in medical journals about perfumes and their ingredients. Websites presented in the Selected Reading section can point the interested reader in this direction.

It follows that you should avoid giving items with irritants such as pine scents as presents to those you know or suspect to have a breathing problem.

The amount of time we are exposed to an irritant is called contact time or exposure time. The longer the contact time, the worse the exposure. Examples include the time we breathe in smoke from cigarettes, fireplaces, and automobile and diesel exhaust.

Exposure time includes inhaling allergens released from our pets. At home it is 100 percent of the time. Exposure time also includes breathing the odors and particles of foods to which we may have an allergy. People with food allergy or asthma can have a clinical reaction just to the smell of the particular food. Big trouble foods this time of the year are nuts and nut roles, fruitcakes, shellfish, and products containing eggs.

Take a little time occasionally to relax and reduce the stress. This is important for your pets as well. Both humans and dogs have allergies and respiratory problems, and getting too excited means a greater number and greater severity of reactions.

In terms of challenge for the lungs and subsequent absorption into the blood of potentially harmful gases, we have no real control over our environment once we are outside the home. Fortunately, the same basic rules apply: cutting back on the amount of time we spend in new clothing, furniture, and especially video and electronic stores. This is where formaldehyde and other chemicals are used for permanent press and fireproofing, and where VOCs from plastics are emitted. Fresh air usually clears the symptoms in a short period of time.

The air in the central walkways of malls is generally much less hazardous to breathe than that of the individual stores. It's the closest thing to fresh air you'll find for awhile, so take frequent breaks and escapes.

If you are buying art supplies or hobby materials for adults or children, ask for nontoxic glues, markers, and other products.

Holiday season cold weather is an asthma trigger. Eighty-five percent of asthmatics have allergic asthma.[25] Exposure to allergens, irritants, and cold in a hurry-up situation can be a recipe for disaster.

Chances are you will be spending time at the home of an elderly person, so be cognizant of the gifts and foods you bring.

Chapter 16

Ventilation in the Home

There are two basic components to a building's ventilation: entry of fresh air and removal of stale air. Both may occur by the same mechanisms. Variations of these will occur in homes, apartments, offices, schools, and other structures.

The entry of air into a home, for example, may occur through a full dozen mechanisms: open or leaky windows, open doors, chimney, plumbing stack, light fixtures, joint between ground floor or basement and the outside, attic hatch, bathroom and kitchen vents, and other areas. The construction of the home will dictate its level of tightness in respect to the amount of normal penetration of outdoor air.

Obviously, we don't want to introduce outdoor pollen, mold, and other particles into the indoor spaces when we ventilate. This issue is addressed in other locations throughout this book.

Normally, we can expect one air change per hour within the home, but this figure may vary as much as tenfold in either direction, depending on whether the home is very tight or very leaky. Obviously, too much either way is not desirable.

Our goal is to remove the sources of pollution and permit fresh air to enter. This involves understanding where the pollution is being generated, doing something about the pollution, and sealing areas of excessive leakage when we can find them. The latter can involve inexpensive weather stripping around doors and windows or attic hatches, tape to seal holes where pipes and wires enter the walls, and ensuring that the chimney damper can close completely. If the home has an attached garage, it is necessary to look for leakage at the sides and bottom of the connecting door. Automotive pollutants are unwelcome guests in any home.

When fresh air is added to a house, its humidity will come along with it. This humidity should be maintained below 60 percent to prevent the proliferation of house-dust mites and mold growth. Inexpensive battery-operated, wall-mounted, or freestanding humidity measuring devices are readily available online, in electronic stores, and in department stores. Ideally, several of these should be purchased at once to place in various areas, including the master bedroom/bath, attic, basement, and main living space. These devices only measure the humidity at the point where they are situated, and not the humidity distant from their placement.

Remember that operation of a central or wall mounted air conditioner or ceiling fan will not remove gaseous pollutants. Coupled with a good-quality filter, the central air conditioner will remove particles as long as the fan is in operation eight hours a day. In many parts of the country, an attic fan will provide good removal of heat and stale air when a window is opened.

Removal of pollution should involve elimination of its source. Air dilution of the space where the source is being generated is helpful. If fragrance products are not used in the home, then that source is completely eliminated. If the bathroom or kitchen stovetop vent fans are used at the right times, then the pollution generated at each of those locations is minimized. This means it will not affect the air quality in the rest of the home, and that you will minimize the need to dilute the indoor air with outdoor air. There may be a difference of as much as seven to fourteen-fold between the amount of fresh air that is required in a home when the kitchen (and bathroom) fan is used.[26] That's a lot of heating and cooling energy to save.

Pollution sources include, but are not limited to, fresh wall paint; press wood products, which all contain formaldehyde; newly varnished or polished furniture and cabinets; new wall paneling, areas where indoor smoking occurs most frequently, living areas for pets, and an attached home garage in need of ventilation.

Installation of a humidistat will permit the automatic activation of fans when the humidity climbs above a certain level.[26] This is especially important in the bathroom, where moisture buildup may help to create an indoor mold problem and an accumulation of truly toxic cleaning and personal care products.

In a home, removal of nonbearing walls can give an aesthetic feeling of openness, and at the same time enable more air mixing and dilution of any pollutants that might otherwise build up in previously compartmented areas of the home. Along those lines, leaving interior doors open when possible will accomplish the same thing on a smaller scale.

There are a number of mechanical devices and ideas available to assist in the addition of fresh air into the home and removal of stale contaminated air. *Wave ventilation units* are available for removal of moisture from basements or crawl spaces, removal of musty odors, and replenishment of fresh air. This makes them a more complete package than a dehumidifier.

Energy recovery ventilators, or ERVs, will significantly reduce the moisture level in a home and reduce the load on the central air-handling system. These remove the moisture from the air and modify the temperature before the air is introduced into the home.

Air-to-air heat exchangers blow warm stale air out of the home and transfer the warmth to incoming fresh air.

Attic ventilation units overcome the tremendous heat buildup in the attic from the outdoor air and reduce moisture buildup. As always, consumers should educate themselves about the natural and mechanical ventilation systems that are the most cost-effective for his home.[27]

Chapter 17

Ventilation in the Office and the Hospital

There are thousands of books, documents, and reports regarding office and hospital ventilation—too many to begin to present a cross-section of their contents. Instead, we will present a peak at a few of the important points that are stressed in those many pages.

Offices

In the office, common sources of pollution include: tobacco smoke that clings to the hair and clothing of smokers, biological organisms, building materials and furnishings, new carpeting and its glue-down mastic, cleaning agents, copy machines, personal care products, and pesticides. The primary areas of concern are the conference room and the copy room. In both cases, the amount of fresh-air ventilation does not compensate for the number of people present, or their personal care products. Additionally, the respiratory irritant ozone is produced in the copy rooms by the machines.

Sick building syndrome, or SBS as noted in the introduction to this section, is the term applied to symptoms without a definable cause. The symptoms include dry mucous membranes and eye, nose, and throat irritation.[28] Sneezing can occur from excessive dust in older buildings, along with a very high concentration of airborne and settled fiber particles from worn carpeting. Many office employees report headaches and a variety of other complaints that can best be defined as esoteric. When they are not weather related, headaches that occur in the office are usually caused by volatile organic compounds (VOCs) rather than by particles. In offices and in schools, workers tend to identify with one another in their suspected medical issues. Mold is at the forefront of these complaints. When no mold contamination is found, some workers find other areas in which to register health complaints.

In my experience, cleaning and maintenance crews are frequently the cause of health-related issues within the office area and the school. The problems here are twofold: use of cleaning products that act as respiratory irritants, and rapid vacuuming and dusting techniques that actually increase the level of airborne particulates rather than reducing it.

Improper airflow balance is common, with the result that stale air can pool in pockets in various areas of the main floor. The use of poor-quality air filters or overloaded air filters is frequently cited as a cause of poor indoor air quality (IAQ). The use of partitions will disturb airflow. Overcrowding an area such as a conference room for an extended time will frequently lead to one or more health-related complaints for the same reasons.

In 1989, ASHRAE published their list of standards for good IAQ. ASHRAE stressed point source control. Where unusual activity is present, they recommend removal of old air and introduction of fresh air. ASHRAE notes that "Providing localized exhaust for these specific sources can result in a reduction of the amount of overall building exhaust ventilation necessary."[29]

Those activities are covered in the chapter regarding ventilation in the home, the section on schools, and a variety of other chapters throughout this book.

In a brief summary of building supply and exhaust locations noted by this author and also presented by the EPA, the information is applicable to most workers.[36]

In offices, the air-handling system should be activated hours before employees enter the building on any given day. Most complaints are logged on a Monday, when the system has been off for two days and the pollutants have increased in concentration.

Neither small nor large offices are immune to the problems. This includes the office in which you might work, as well as multistoried buildings of all types, including army command centers on military bases.

Hospitals

The same issues that plague office buildings in general also plague hospitals.

Building design and maintenance in older (and possibly newer) hospitals serve as examples of what not to do: return air supply vents are located in close proximity to exhaust vents on the roof; central air-handling filters are changed well beyond the point of their collapse to save money; fresh air supplies are located near the diesel truck loading dock; and exhaust fans are not utilized in the areas where they are most needed due to the presence of chemical supplies and latex-laden cornstarch from gloves. These areas include hematology, pediatrics, microbiology, and X-ray film development. The good news is that there has been a strong move to avoid the use of latex gloves in clinical settings.

Additionally, the hundreds of alcohol wipes used daily can raise the indoor level of volatile organic compounds to seven hundred ppm, including emergency, pediatrics, microbiology, and hematology. (A baseline VOC level should range from 0.0 to 0.5 ppm.) Open trash containers are common, and foot-operated containers may not be in overabundance. It is these same areas where cornstarch-laden antigens from latex gloves might be found in high concentrations.

Remodeling efforts are frequently a problem when proper containment between old and new wings is not maintained. A wide variety of disease-causing particulates, including pathogenic *Aspergillus spp.* mold, may be present above drop-ceiling portions of the old wing. These can travel to a wing where chemotherapy is in progress, with serious consequences for the patients.

Endnotes

1. Ott, R. 1998. Everyday exposure to toxic pollutants. *Scientific American*. Feb.

2. Spengler, J.D., J.M. Samet and J.F. McCarthy. 2001. *Indoor Air Quality Handbook*. Pesticides. McGraw-Hill, New York.

3. Agarwal, M.K., et al. 1984. Airborne ragweed allergens: association with various particle sizes and short ragweed plant parts. *J Allergy Clin Immunol*. Nov;74(5)687-93.

4. Foliage or Clean Air Council. 1990. Indoor plants are clean air machines.*Gardening*. June 1:11.

5. NASA Center for Aerospace Information. 2007. Plants clean air and water for indoor environments. Dec. **www.sti.nasa.gov**.

6. Blazovsky,C. 2004 Plants make a healthy home. *Our Toxic Times*, (Newsletter for the Chemical Injury Information Network) Great Falls, Mo. Oct.

7. Burge, H. 1982. Evaluation of indoor plantings as allergen exposure sources. *J Allergy Clin Immunol*. 70:2,101-108.

8. Olkowski, W., S. Daar, and H. Olkowski. 1993. *Common-Sense Pest Control. Least Toxic Solutions for Your Home, Garden, Pets and Community*. By Taunton Press, Newtown, Conn.

9. Ware, G.W. 1996. *Complete Guide to Pest Control: With and Without Chemicals* (3rd Ed.) Thomson Publications, Fresno, Calif.

10. Green Leaf Mapping and Control Systems. 1998. Vacuum and soap kill insects on plants. Reprinted from *USA Today Magazine*, 126:10.

11. USDA. 2006. Soy ink superior degradability. Nov. 3 published in *Agricultural Research Magazine*, Jan. 1995.

12. Printing Responsibly. 2009. *Soy Inks*. (Soyseal). **www.soy-growers.com/resources/soyink**.

13. Ibid.

14. EPA. 2009. *An introduction to indoor air quality: Sources of combustion products.* Jan 15. **www.epa.gov/iaq/combust**.

15. NFPA. 1997. *Fire Protection Handbook.* 18th Ed. Quincy, Mass. National Fire Protection Assoc.

16. Wallace,L., et al. 1987 Emissions of volatile organic compounds from building materials and consumer products. *Atmospheric Environ.* 21:2,385-393.

17. Reed Business Information. 2008. Roll up the red carpet and lay down tiles. *Building Product News.* Oct.

18. Salzmann, A. and J. Silberner. 1989. When each day is a sick day. *U.S. News & World Report.* March

19. U.S. Department of Health and Human Services. 2000. NIOSH Hazard Review: *Carbonless Copy Paper.* Centers for Disease Control and Prevention. Dec.

20. Office of Environmental Health Hazard Assessment (OEHHA). 2007. Guideline for the safe use of art and craft materials. *Childrens Health.* Dec. **www.oehha.ca.gov/education/art/artguide**.

21. Zaide, S. et al. 2007. Multi-organ toxicity and death following acute unintentional inhalation of paint thinner fumes. *Clin Toxicol.* March 45:3,287-289.

22. Brody, J. 1994. Personal Health. *The New York Times.* March.

23. National Institute of Deafness and other communication disorders. 2008. *How Loud is Too Loud?* April. **www.nidcd.nih.gov/health/hearing/ruler.asp**.

24. Galen Carol udo. Decibel (Loudness) Comparison Chart. Study by M. Chasin, *FAAA Centre for Human Performance and Health.*

25. Children's Hospital of Wisconsin. 2009. Cold weather can trigger asthma. Children's Hospital and Health System. **www.chw.org/display/PPF/DocID/33019/Nav/1/router.asp**

26. Coffel, S. and K. Feiden. 1991. A Proper airing: The Science of Ventilation. *Indoor Pollution.* Ballantine Books, New York.

27. Stewart, B.R. Agricultural Extension Services. Texas A&M University. Attic Ventilation for Homes. **www.factsfacts.com/MyHomeRepair/ventilation**.

28. EPAA. Ventilation and Air Quality in Offices. Fact Sheet. *Air and Radiation*. Document 402-F-94-003 (6609J).

29. ASHRAE. 1989. Ventilation for Acceptable Indoor Air Quality Standards 62-1989.

OEHHA and NIOSH websites provide a great deal of information regarding a wide variety of health hazards that the consumer encounters in daily life including air pollution, food and water safety and workplace hazards.

In addition to the above references, the reader is invited to read John Bower's book on The Healthy Home, as referenced in the Suggested Reading portion of this book.

Section 7

Pets and Critters

From a number of standpoints, pets contribute to their masters' allergic symptoms. Antigens (allergens) from pets include their hair and fur, skin cells (dander), saliva, urine from cat litter boxes, the litter itself (which becomes airborne and is also tracked throughout the entire home, school, or workplace), and the indoor tracking of allergens from out-of-doors. Mammalian pets, specifically cats and dogs, are among the worst offenders because of their fur, their numbers, and their frequent indoor and outdoor sojourns and contamination of their bedding. Because cat allergens are more universal in their presence and because they are potent allergens, they are more important than dog allergens.

The presence of insects is also a universal problem. These include cockroaches, mites, ticks, fleas, and their body parts, including their feces. The scientist needs only to peer through the microscope to see these insect particles that are in our air. Their removal requires preventive action accompanied with diligent housecleaning and the use of non toxic pesticides.

Chapter 1
Pets and Your Children's Allergies

The majority of parents of allergic children believe that the pet is expensive, unnecessary for their child's happiness, harmful to the health, not clean, and a carrier of allergens. They are quite aware of the problems that the pet may create in the household, and all feel that their child's allergy is more important than their pet. Given this, very few parents—or children, for that matter—feel that removal of the pet would affect the child psychologically, even though the pet is considered part of the family. Given that parents of allergic and asthmatic children understand that their child is reactive, the question becomes, why do they maintain the pets in the home? Part of the answer is wrapped in emotional and sentimental involvement with the animal.

This complex topic has been studied and reported on in a number of medical and veterinarian surveys. Most professionals agree that there are several reasons for the retention of pets in the homes of allergic (asthmatic) children. One reason is tied in with parental resentment toward the child because of the illness, which incorporates visits that involve time and money related to medical expenses for the child. Everyone shares in the inconvenience of seeing the doctor, the missed schoolwork and changed living patterns, and not being able to do what you want when you want to do it. In many ways this is no different than the resentment felt toward elderly persons living in the home.

In addition, some parents had more confidence in the opinions expressed by their veterinarian than those of their allergist. This is because many allergists advocate complete removal of the pet from the home, while the vet is more sympathetic. Parents felt that the vet could more easily relate to the pet as a loved one in the family and try to strike compromise solutions with family members so that they would not have to give up this loved one. According to the surveys, some parents confide to their veterinarian and pet store owners that they believe the child will overcome the illness eventually, even if the pet is allowed to remain.

Finally, some parents did not like anyone telling them what to do in their home, including their doctor.

There is no substitute for removal of an allergen source and sound medical advice. However, compromise solutions include maintaining the pet in isolated areas of the home or exclusively out-of-doors. Certainly, it should not be permitted in the child's bedroom. Some parents will have shaggy pets like cocker spaniels, Persian cats, or Angora rabbits shaved down, according to some pet store owners. Regardless of the route you choose, they are still potentially allergenic. Dog hair is not necessarily considered to be an allergen because hair is too large a particle to be inhaled, but it does contain the dander to which the allergens attach.

Chapter 2

Cats

Depending on where you live, 15 to 40 percent of allergic people are allergic to cats or dogs. Allergy to cats is about twice as common as it is to dogs. While there are no hypoallergenic cats, males produce less allergen than do females, and neutered males produce less allergen than do non-neutered males.[1]

Cat hair is not allergenic unto itself because we don't inhale the hair. Rather, cat allergen is produced by the sebaceous (oil) glands. It is stored primarily on the surface of the skin and fur, with its greatest concentration at the hair roots. Hair is involved to the extent that the cats lick the hair, and the sebaceous (oil) glands coat it with antigen as well. The highly potent and long-lived allergen is gradually spread to the tip of the shaft, where it may become airborne and produce allergic respiratory symptoms.

Cat allergen is comprised of two small and potent protein molecules, called sticky proteins. They're attracted to soft furnishings such as the sofa, armchair, bedding, and carpets. The allergen is present in settled dust and air samples from homes without cats. In fact, the antigen is so universal that it has been found in every building where it has been sought, including newly built homes, shopping malls, doctors' offices, and even hospitals. Presumably people track it in, or bring it in on clothing and possessions.

People who are allergic to cats can react within fifteen to thirty minutes after exposure,[2] and possibly within seconds.

They usually experience a rapid onset of symptoms as soon as they enter a room where a cat is present.

Cat antigen takes six months to three years to disappear from a home, even after the cat is gone And no cleaning is performed. It is in its highest amount on the bed and mattress or soft furnishings that the cat frequents.

A good, thorough housecleaning and scrubbing will significantly remove this highly allergenic protein that sticks to soft furnishings and adheres to walls, although I have found that there can be a clinically high amount of cat protein three years after the cat(s) has been removed (i.e., 10 micrograms of protein per gram of dust).

It is debatable if washing a cat will remove the antigens from it. However, even if it works, the allergens will regenerate within a short time. A freestanding or even central high-efficiency particulate air (HEPA) filter (air purifier) will not make a difference. This is because the antigen (allergen) is being produced as fast as it is being removed. With the cat still present, the current thinking is that it's impossible to remove enough of the allergen to lessen the onset of clinical symptoms.

The interested reader may wish to follow some recommended measures to reduce their exposure level to their pet *in the hopes* that they might reduce their symptoms.

» Keep the pet out of the bedroom, and restrict it to as few rooms in the home as possible.

» Allergic individuals should not pet, hug, or kiss their pets because of allergens on the pet's fur or saliva.

» Keep pets off soft furnishings.

» Ensure that litter boxes are placed away from air return registers or fresh air supplies.

» Wear a protective mask when grooming your pet and remove clothing after grooming.

» After grooming, wash your face and hands.
» Use high-efficiency vacuum cleaner bags or vacuum cleaners with HEPA filters.

Cat litter particles—containing cat urine, cat feces, and harmful fragrance (toluene)—are readily recognizable under the microscope. According to my measurements, they can number as many as ten thousand per cubic yard (or meter) in areas of the home distant from the litter box. This is considered to be an extremely high number and rivals outdoor pollen and spore counts throughout many areas of the country. Change the litter box frequently. Otherwise, cats will track their "litter business" all over the house, even onto kitchen counters.

Chapter 3

Cat Stats

Approximately six million Americans are allergic to cats.

Fifty percent of all allergic people are allergic to cats.

Cats are more likely than any other animal to cause allergy problems.

Thirty percent of all asthmatics are allergic to cats and may have an asthma attack when exposed to cat allergen.

Approximately one-third of homes in the United States have at least one cat, for a total cat population of over fifty million.

One-third of those allergic to cats continue to keep them at home.

Carpets, mattresses, and soft furnishings are the major reservoirs of cat allergen in the home.

Cat allergen is often present in houses that cats have never entered.

Due to the small size of cat allergen particles (2.5 to 10 microns), they remain airborne for long periods of time.

People allergic to cats develop symptoms rapidly upon entering a house with cats, in contrast to those who are allergic to dust.

House-dust mite, cat, and cockroach allergens are the three main indoor allergens in North America. Exposure to any one of these in early childhood may lead to the development of asthma.

A significant amount of cat allergen can linger in a mattress for more than three years after the cat has been removed. It is advisable to make use of impermeable mattress encasings in any house where a cat lives or has lived.

In a house with a cat, aggressive cleaning, good ventilation, and removal of soft furnishings can dramatically reduce levels of allergen.

Chapter 4
Cat Antigen Cleanup

Because the highly allergenic proteins have a predilection for soft furnishings, it was once thought that the only way to get rid of them was to wash the home with a 3 percent tannic acid solution, or to get rid of the soft furnishings or the cats.

Two-thirds of people allergic to cats do not even own one. Homes with cats have from ten to one hundred times the amount of cat allergen compared with homes that have no cats, and 25 percent of the allergen is in particles less than 2.5 microns in size, small enough to enter the deeper lung spaces and cause the rapid onset of symptoms within minutes.

Larger particles greater than five microns can still induce symptoms after longer periods of time, that is, hours later. This reaction is not only likely to be much more serious, but it will also leave the lungs sensitive to many other nonallergic triggers such as cold air, exercise, and cigarette smoke, which in turn makes the person more sensitive to cat allergen—a vicious cycle. Eventually, if this cycle continues, there may be irreversible damage to the airways.

There is much more allergen in rooms where the air is disturbed. This means that even if you have a freestanding HEPA filtration air purifier in a given room, the cat allergen will always be airborne and respirable. This is because the clean air that is coming out of the unit will disturb the settled allergen almost as much as the filter will remove the allergen. In other words, a freestanding HEPA filtration unit cannot be expected to reduce the exposure level of occupants to cat antigen or reduce the number and severity of symptoms.

Most homes have only 0.5 changes of fresh air or fewer per hour. At ten changes per hour the amount of allergen will be reduced. With that much fresh air, even though there will be more turbulence, the allergen will be carried outside.

A water filter vacuum cleaner may not be suitable for patients with cats, because its use results in a sharp increase in the allergen associated with fine droplets created by the machine.

In addition to genetic factors, exposure to high levels of dust mite, cat, or cockroach allergen in early childhood may contribute to the development of asthma. It is well documented that people with immediate hypersensitivity to cat allergen will, at some time, develop acute asthmatic symptoms.

The preferred method of symptom management is to reduce the patient's exposure to cat allergen through environmental control.

If you insist on keeping your cat, try to eliminate soft furnishings and limit the pet's territory within the home. It is advisable to cover your mattresses and pillows with impermeable covers. This is true, in any case, if you have allergic asthma.

Good ventilation can also dramatically reduce the amount of cat allergen in the home. Unfortunately, modern homes that are energy-efficient, with a low rate of fresh-air exchange, trap the smallest particles of cat allergen inside, where they either remain airborne or settle on soft furnishings. If the particles settle on soft furnishings, they can easily become airborne again when they associate with dust particles.

Vacuum cleaners need filters to prevent cat allergen in the carpet from escaping through the exhaust. HEPA vacuum filters are more useful after the carpet has been vigorously cleaned.

Be aware that vacuuming a home with the windows closed will liberate a tremendous amount of cat antigen at face level with all but the best vacuuming systems.

It is common to find patients sensitive to cats who have never lived with a cat. These people became allergic to cats through a variety of means. Some of these include becoming sensitized through contact with formaldehyde or common outdoor air pollutants.

Any measurable amount of cat antigen might be clinically important, and it is obvious that total avoidance is not possible. You should carefully consider the need for medications.

If you are going to remove your cat from your environment and aggressively clean your home, it might be a good idea to get a new mattress as well. And don't forget to clean your ductwork.

Many people would rather keep their cats and suffer from allergies. For them, getting a professional to wash and groom their pets has its own rewards. For those whose affliction is serious enough, however, removal of the cat from the home, together with a serious housecleaning, is still the best method of indoor cat allergen reduction.

Chapter 5

Dogs

Dog allergen is very specific to dogs and does not cross-react with cat, bird, cockroach, or dust-mite allergen. Dog allergen is probably present in half the homes in this country. Chances are you have some around, even if you don't own a dog.

Skin cells of dogs are allergenic. Long-hair dogs have been reported to be less allergenic than short-hair breeds because long-hair dogs shed fewer skin cells into the air.[3] This is relatively unimportant other than in a scientific sense, however. It's tough for even one hair to get into the respiratory tract to cause an allergic reaction. If we analyze the air of homes where dogs are present, we do not find a lot of airborne hairs because they are heavy and settle out onto surfaces. What we do find is a tremendous number of skin cells throughout the entire home, especially in the room that contains the dog's bed.

From the human standpoint it is important to have your pet groomed and well cared for to maximize its health and minimize your own exposure to allergenic animal dander (skin cells) and hair. Regular care keeps the coat healthy and reduces the shedding. (This may not make any difference as far as cats are concerned, because it is not their dander that is allergenic.)

A person who is sensitive to dogs will probably react to any breed. However, if you are looking for a breed that is less allergenic to humans, try a poodle or a terrier. These dogs shed less hair and dander than long-hair breeds.

Chapter 6

Birds

There are millions of pet birds in the United States. Most of them are parakeets, canaries, and finches, with lesser numbers of cockatiels and parrots.[4] There are also a number of diseases that both wild and cultivated birds transmit to humans. Allergenic birds include chickens, turkeys, starlings, and others. The diseases they transmit go by the exotic names of cryptococcosis, histoplasmosis, Newcastle disease, cryptosporidiosis, salmonellosis, and psittacosis.

The antigen from domestic birds is responsible for a variety of rare respiratory ailments. The most common of these are allergic rhinitis, asthma, and hypersensitivity pneumonitis.

Because allergy to birds is rare, the decision to keep avian pets out of the home should be made on a case-by-case basis.

Source of bird antigens

When bird antigens are a problem, it is their droppings that are the main troublemaker, though there may be others.

Birds shed tiny feathers that become airborne. However, these are not inhaled to the extent that they become an issue.

Certain birds such as doves (including pigeons), cockatoos, and cockatiels produce a powder on their wings that may be allergenic. These particles can be readily found in the air within many if not most homes and buildings, and outdoors. A great deal of this powder originates from pigeons, which are a nuisance due to their roosting on roofs and attic spaces. In certain areas of the country, other doves or quail may be more prevalent.

The powder serves as a waterproofing agent for the birds. Outdoors, the concentration of the powder varies greatly, but indoors, the level can be as high as two thousand per cubic yard (meter) of air or more.

The size of these powder particles ranges from two to ten microns, with virtually all particles in the three-micron size range. Therefore, they are all respirable.

Location of bird antigens

Pigeons on the roofs of buildings can roost around fresh air intakes. They are a problem because fragments of their droppings are pulled into the building's ductwork. Wild bird excrement deposited outside the home may be a source of antigen in the home if it is tracked indoors on shoes.

Fortunately, while cats and dogs are free to contaminate the entire home, pet birds are generally contained in a cage in a particular room. Bird antigen from feces is found predominantly in the area where the bird is kept and in lesser amounts distant from the pet. This makes sense, as the bird stays in one location. The exception to this is when the bird spends a great deal of time away from the cage in other areas of the house. Then the particles from the powder on their wings remain airborne indefinitely because of their light weight.

Longevity of bird antigens

Like cat antigen, bird antigen from feces will remain in the home long after the pet is gone and is found primarily in the soft furnishings and deep-pile carpets. The latter will store the most antigen.

Powder particles are airborne much longer, so clean the

cage weekly if you suspect there might be a health issue related to your pet birds.

Antigens associated with a bird can remain in the home for as long as eighteen months or more after the bird is removed. This means that clinical symptoms can persist during that period.

Solutions

If you have a sensitivity to birds, here are some tips that you should consider:

» Clean your bird's room two to three times weekly.

» If possible, keep your bird in a room that has wooden or tile floors. This will help you keep the room clean. It will also prevent the spread of antigen elsewhere in the home. Keeping the door closed to the bird's room will help reduce the level of airborne antigen when coupled with an air purifier designated for that room.

» Clean the cage at least once a week.

» It is unfortunate, but studies have shown that normal cleaning of carpets does not remove the antigen. However, deep steam cleaning may help because its heat can destroy the protein antigen.

» Remove your shoes when entering the home so as not to track in antigens from wild bird excrement.

» Do not kiss the bird.

Chapter 7

Horses

Tens of millions of Americans own, ride, or come in contact with horses on a regular basis.

Some people are highly allergic to all horses. For years, people have been telling each other and telling their doctors that they are allergic to some horse breeds and not to others. The investigation into this matter became a major study.

Are some breeds of horses more allergenic than others?

If we compare different horse breeds, including the Swedish halfbreed, Haflinger, Arabian thoroughbred, bashkir curly, Russian bashkir, and American trotting horse, we find that there are no antigens that are specific to a certain breed.[5] In other words, if you are allergic to one breed of horse, then you are allergic to them all.

The dander of long-hair horses, such as bashkir, is just as allergenic as the dander from short-hair horses, such as Arabians and thoroughbreds. The end result is that a person will react with less severity and with less frequency to long-hair breeds because their skin cells do not escape as readily. This helps explain why many persons report that they are not allergic to long-hair horses.[5]

Chapter 8

Pets Have Allergies Too

<hr>

Dogs react to allergens, but in a different way than humans. The difference is that humans sneeze and dogs scratch.

Allergies in dogs are more severe when they begin at an early age. When sensitivities develop, they can be to pollen, mold, house dust, food, chemicals, insect bites, or any number of other substances. Similar to humans, dogs inherit the tendency to be allergic.[6]

Respiratory allergy in dogs is commonly manifested by severe itching and scratching of the skin. This causes them to lick and scratch and bite the paws. Other symptoms may include sneezing, coughing, tearing, or diarrhea. If your dog starts to scratch at the same time each year, he or she may be suffering from a skin allergy due to breathing tree pollen during the spring and summer months, spring and fall for grasses, and spring and fall for ragweed and other weed pollens, depending on where in the country you live. A high percentage of dogs will develop clinical allergic symptoms at one time or another.

Reactions to mold can be seasonal, as well. Allergic reactions to mold also occur indoors in the damp basement, attic, or in an area where a carpet or other surface is providing nutrition for the mold. In this case, see if the pet's initial reactions occur in a particular room. Also watch for licking at a runny nose, rubbing an itchy face on the carpet, and other symptoms mentioned above for clues to an allergy problem.

Respiratory allergy in dogs can be confused with flea and tick allergy and irritations to the eyes and ears. This occurs most commonly in Dalmatians, poodles, cocker spaniels, golden retrievers, and terriers, but all breeds can be affected.[6]

Food allergies in dogs and cats are not uncommon, especially with today's processed and preserved foods. Food allergies tend to occur year-round rather than seasonally, as with pollen and mold. Severe itching is very common here, and one must rule out allergy to other coat irritants.

Many people will use their own shampoo on their pet. This practice may dry the animal's skin, as its shampoo for humans is not balanced for the pet's skin in terms of relative acidity and other factors. Check with your vet on this issue.

What can the pet owner do to determine if the pet has an allergy?

According to veterinarians, the first step is to educate yourself as to the signs and symptoms of pet allergies compared with other animal disorders. Then do some detective work. Perhaps lice or ticks are present in the coat. These can also cause the itching. Is there a rash around the snout due to sensitivity to a new food dish? Are there new plants in bloom, or do you have a home with a lawn? Like humans, pets can react to the chemicals in a new carpet; they may have difficulty breathing, or their eyes may tear. This is also true when they are exposed to cigarette smoke.

Most veterinarians will perform allergy testing on your pet, either skin tests or blood tests.

If you determine that an allergy is present in your dog, and you believe it is manifest in the skin, a bath will be helpful. Use an anti-allergy shampoo and bathe the animal in cool water. Warm water may irritate the skin condition. Leave the shampoo in contact with the skin for ten to fifteen minutes, or as per veterinarian recommendations. This will reduce the inflammation and help to rehydrate the skin. After rinsing the shampoo, follow the treatment with a moisturizer (no fragrances please). For treatment of dogs, tar-sulfur shampoos are available with a prescription.

Be careful. Shampoos can be fatal to cats, as cats are more sensitive than dogs to most medications and treatments.[7] Again, check with your vet or pet groomer for proper shampoos to use on your pet.

Dietary supplements will help. Recommended are Omega 3 and omega 6 fatty acids; the liquid works better than the powder. These anti-inflammatory fatty acids will affect the sheen of the coat from the inside out and will serve to reduce the itching and scratching. Reduction of scratching means that your own exposure to the allergenic dander and hair will also be minimized. This is an important consideration.

Once the results of a sensitivity test are known, you may be able to provide desensitization shots to your pet at home.

Similar to the circumstance of human allergies, your vet may call for more aggressive treatment of the pet's problem. This treatment may include the injection of corticosteroids. Also, ask your vet about ticks and fleas. Treatment by a grooming shop is less expensive, but may cause problems to your pet until you can identify the specific problem.

Chapter 9

House-Dust Mites

House-dust mites are a problem throughout most of the world. Each mite sheds about twenty fecal pellets daily, and it is these fecal pellets that are allergenic. Because they are microscopic, they can readily enter the lungs. Dust mite feces are among the world's greatest respiratory allergens, along with ragweed and grass pollen, cat allergen, and cockroach allergen.

Mites belong to the same family as ticks and spiders. There are forty-six species of mites, of which thirteen have been found in house dust. However, only two to four of these species are of the most concern to the allergic and asthmatic population.

In the United States the two prominent species are *Dermatophagoides pteronyssinus* and *D. farinae.*

Mites are so small that a dozen of them would fit in the period at the end of this sentence. Under the microscope they look similar to crabs.

Mites probably adapted to the ecological habitat of the human household from the nests of various birds and mammals, where they are most commonly found. They eat skin cells that humans and pets shed, as well as bacteria and fungi. They do not bite, but their fecal matter and body parts are extremely small, respirable, and highly allergenic. It is the feces that science focuses upon.

Mites do not obtain their water from their diet—they extract it from the air. Therefore, they do well in a more humid environment.

In the home, mites are most numerous in overstuffed chairs and sofas and in the carpet next to these areas. Mattresses and blankets are also involved in the harboring of the creatures; spring mattresses harbor more mites than the foam type. The bed offers the mites warmth, food, humidity, and protection. A microclimate that exists in the mattress for up to sixteen hours a day can be vastly different than the climate of the home as a whole. The mattress remains warmer and more humid due to the presence of sleeping bodies.

Draperies can be added to the list of places where mites congregate. Additionally, soft toys are likely to be an important source of mite allergens in childhood asthma.

As noted above, mites prefer moisture to dryness. They prefer an indoor relative humidity (RH) of 65 to 75 percent and a room temperature of 72 to 79 degrees Fahrenheit. These are also excellent conditions for mold growth. Immature mites can become dormant with cooler temperatures and less humidity, surviving for months until the moisture level increases again. Mature mites cannot survive when the RH is below 50 percent. Thus, mites are common in more humid climates of the country and the world.

Despite similar construction, each home is quite different as far as the number of mites. One hundred mites per gram are considered to be at the threshold of sensitivity. (A packet of sugar weighs a gram.) Few homes have a number as low as this, however. Most have between five hundred and two thousand per gram of dust.[8]

Here are some suggestions for reducing mite allergens in the home:

» Replace feather pillows with synthetics.
» Wash bedding weekly in water hotter than 130 degrees Fahrenheit (54 degrees Celsius) to kill live mites. A 5

percent solution of household bleach will also kill mites
(1:20 dilution).

» Encase your mattress and box spring in plastic.

» Vacuum the mattress, base of the bed, bed frame, rugs,
carpets, and upholstered furniture regularly. Carpets
will have a higher humidity level, in general, although
mites are less frequently found at carpet edges.

» Wet-mop the baseboards or at least the area where the
floor meets the walls when possible and be sure to pay
attention to these areas while vacuuming. Attention
should also be paid to the wiping of windowsills.

» The use of air-conditioning, dehumidifiers, and air filtration devices all serve to decrease, but not eliminate,
the mite population.[9] This is also true of vacuum cleaners.

Chapter 10
Cockroaches

As mentioned elsewhere in this book, indoor allergens and other respiratory irritants (particles and gases) are known to have a greater impact on the asthmatic population than those same substances found out-of-doors. This is due to their higher concentration in the indoor environment and the fact that the occupants spend more time indoors.

In an allergen-rich environment, the aeroallergens prime the bronchial system to respond readily to such factors as changes in the weather, cooking smells, or insects and insect sprays.

One of the most important indoor allergens in the inner city areas is the cockroach. It is similar to the house-dust mite in that the antigen is composed of feces, but its body parts are also allergenic. The cockroach antigen is at least as potent as that of ragweed, and the problem becomes worse with continued exposure.

The cockroach problem is most common among the lower socioeconomic groups, but these insects can also be rampant in middle-income apartment complexes. The species most commonly found as a household pest in the United States is *Blatella germanica* (the German cockroach).

Studies have shown that for the cockroach to become a medical problem, there must be a significant infestation,[10] although some people might consider one roach to fit that requirement.

The inhalation of anti-cockroach spray in the home or apartment can be potentially hazardous to the respiratory health of many people. The residence should not be entered until the spray has had a chance to completely settle out of the air, at which point fresh air should be utilized to flush the home of pesticide.

Unless covered, the spray will be absorbed by furnishings and bedding. These areas should be covered prior to spraying, although typically the roaches are found in the kitchen, beneath the refrigerator, and in the cupboards, where they look for food.

Fortunately, the most basic anti-roach procedure is also the least expensive—-boric acid or borax.[11] (Please see chapter on Borax in Section 13.)

Endnotes

1. Adelglass,J. 2009.*Cat & Dog Allergy*. Ear Nose and Throat Testing & Treatment Center. Feb. **www.entdocs.org/catallergy**

2. Asthma and Allergy Foundation of America. 2005. Pet Allergies. (google aafa pet allergies)

3. More, D. 2009. Dog Allergy. Health's Disease and Condition about Allergies. Feb. **www.allergies.about.com/od/specificallergens/a/dogallergy.htm?p=1**

4. Drisdelle, R. 2008. The most popular pet birds. *Pet Birds.* Feb. **www.pet-birds.suite101.com/article.cfm/the_most_popularpet_birds**

5. Steinman, H. 2003. *Allergens within epidermals and animal proteins.* ImmunoCAP In Vitrosight.

6. Bren, L. 2004. Is your pet itching for relief. *FDA Consumer Report.* U.S. Food and Drug Administration. July-Aug. **www.fad.gov/fdac/features/2004/404_pets.html**

7. Bren, L. 2001. Taking the bite out of fleas and ticks. *FDA Consumer Magazine.* July.

8. Babe, K. et al. 1995. House dust mite prevalence in the rooms and hallways of a tertiary care hospital. *Clinical aspects of Allergic Disease.* Jan 0091-6749/95.

9. Ellingson, A. et al. 1995. The prevalence of *Dermatophagoides* mite allergen in Colorado homes utilizing central evaporative coolers. *J Allergy Clin Immunol* Oct. 96:4

10. Bernstein, J. 2008. Cockroach Allergen and Avoidance. Net Wellness Consumer Health Information. Dec. www.Netwellness.org/healthtopics/allergies/cockroach.cfm.

11. Potter, M. 2007. Cockroach Elimination. U.K. Cooperative Extension Service. College of Agriculture ENTFACT-614 www.ca.uky.edu/entomology/entfacts/ef614.asp.

The Asthma and Allergy Foundation of America is a not-for-profit organization founded in 1953 and is the leading patient organization for people with asthma and allergies and the oldest asthma and allergy patient group in the world. The mission of AAFA's Web site is to provide online access to AAFA's reliable, validated asthma and allergy information and tools to families, patients, parents, healthcare providers, policymakers and others.

As is true throughout this text, exact website designations are frequently not needed if one wishes to research a topic, since the topic may simply be entered into a search engine to obtain many sources.

Section 8

Machines and Devices in the Home

The manufacture of devices that affect our indoor air in one manner or another has become a very large industry. In many cases, the products seem like they should work and our common sense tells us that they will. In other cases, science says otherwise and tells us that they work if we think they will, but there is no actual proof that they will. Another way of saying this is that blind studies often demonstrate similar results when comparing control groups with experimental groups. Let's look at few of the most common types that are used for air "purification and cleaning."

A major problem in the study of the health vs. device issue is that it is virtually impossible to establish an experiment to demonstrate that there is a clinical benefit to the user. In essence, the only thing that can be shown is that there may or may not be a reduction of particles or volatile gases. This does not necessarily translate to better health.

I would be a neglectful microbiologist if I did not remind the reader to pay attention to the transmission of viruses, via these machines and devices. The reader may be familiar with the cautions regarding the necessity to hand-wash after touching shopping cart handles and checkout isle railings. Indeed, children have a propensity to put their mouths on these railings. Within the home, when one or more family members is ill, the transmission of viruses is easily accomplished though the handling of door knobs, refrigerator and microwave door handles, and the front and sides of these units, and a wide variety of common-use objects, followed by hand-to-mouth-or-nose contact.

Frequent hand-washing is recommended as a daily practice to minimize exposure to viruses.

Chapter 1

Ozone

Appliances will produce ozone to varying degrees when they are motorized or have electricity associated with them. These appliances include older central electronic air purifiers, refrigerators, blenders, clothes and hair dryers, and irons.

Ozone is an oxygen molecule with an additional atom of oxygen added. The extra atom gives it a negative charge, and it quickly degrades to oxygen, with the extra atom free to react with other molecules in air or in water.

The Environmental Protection Agency has worked with other federal agencies to assess the scientific literature regarding the use of ozone in the home. Many of the legitimate peer-reviewed articles go back nearly one hundred years. Here is the latest assessment of their findings, available online from the EPA.[1]

The air concentration of ozone at ground level is between 10-25 parts per 10 and 25 billion parts per billion (ppb). Smoggy cities will have ten times this amount. Ozone is considered to be toxic at 60 ppb, while the World Health Organization standard sets 50 ppb as a limit. Children are more sensitive than adults to ozone and will have decreased lung function at the 60 ppb level. Most manufacturers of ozone generators recommend that they be used in the 30 to 50 ppb range. The Occupational Safety and Health Administration (OSHA) limit exposure in the workplace to 100 ppb.

Importantly, no agency of the federal government has approved the use of ozone-generating machines sold as air cleaners.[2]

The response to the odor can vary greatly from person to person.

The issues:

» Does ozone remove odors, and if so, what kinds of odors does it remove?

» Why do some people swear by the use of ozone to rid their homes of air-quality problems?

» Does ozone within a home or building actually reduce the incidence of allergy and asthma?

» Why is ozone considered to be unsafe, and at what level is it unsafe?

» Ozone is promoted as a biocide to kill mold and bacteria. Will it do this?

» How does ozone treatment compare with an air purifier for removal of respiratory irritants?

According to the World Health Organization there are over three hundred chemicals that can be identified in the air of the average home. Both laboratory and in-home experiments have found that ozone reacts with only a certain small class of these chemicals. What is created from the reaction is not pure carbon dioxide and water, as many dealers and manufacturers of in-home ozone machines claim, but formaldehyde. The level of formaldehyde can actually increase with ozone treatment, and ozone will not react with this gas.

In addition to the production of formaldehyde, the chemicals that ozone does react with may produce odorless free radicals that may be more hazardous than the original odor-causing agents. This is the nature of many, if not most, free radicals. Thus, when reacting with volatile organic compounds (VOCs), ozone produces a number of new compounds. The total concentration of VOCs can actually increase in the home in the presence of ozone.

Do odors decrease with the use of ozone? Yes, say researchers. The reason is fourfold. First, if the consumer believes the odor is decreased, then so it will be. Second, ozone is a classic masking agent, and the pungent odor of ozone covers (obscures) the other odors. Third, many researchers have found that ozone affects the odor receptors in the nose, inhibiting our ability to smell. This is why some people swear by the use of ozone—they can't smell the odor anymore. Finally, it may cause the breakdown of chemicals that do have an odor into free radicals that do not have an odor, but which may pose their own health problem.

What kinds of odors doesn't ozone work against at the concentrations that are tolerable to humans? These include tobacco smoke, detergents, waxes, cleaners, and scented room air fresheners. Some literature states that even at a high level, it would take between 880 and 4,400 years to remove household odors with the use of ozone.

How do we know these things? Because we can monitor the exact chemicals with which we started in a home, and with the use of instruments, find out that most of them are still there after ozone treatment. They just can't be smelled.

Does ozone treatment reduce the incidence of allergy and asthma? Research suggests that low ozone concentrations can increase sensitivity of the airways to allergens and aggravate asthma.[3]

Some scientists believe that the EPA should tighten standards on ozone exposure. Some manufacturers of ozone machines are in trouble with the Federal Trade Commission for making false claims of health benefits for the following reasons. First, the FTC doesn't recognize ozone treatment as a legitimate air-cleaning method and does not endorse any type of air cleaners. Second, the policy statement of the American Society for Heating, Refrigeration, and Air Conditioning Engineers (ASHRAE) states that, while ozone can oxidize odors in water, the level required to do this in air would be harmful to building occupants: "The major effect of ozone generators is to reduce sensitivity of the sense of smell, rather than reduce actual odor concentrations."[4,5,6]

Why is ozone under attack from virtually all quarters, except for true believers and those who sell the units that generate the gas? The answer is that, reportedly, those who support the use of ozone for in-home use do not come up with hard data that is contrary to published scientific findings.

Ozone has been used for years as post-fire odor-control. The level of ozone used for this purpose is extremely high and is not compatible with human habitation. (Please refer to the chapter on house fires.)

In summary, I have reviewed scores of scientific papers that point to the germicidal power of ozone. These papers have common problems: the studies are conducted in laboratory conditions; the concentrations that are used are above the human tolerance level; some discuss the use of ozone in water, not in air; and there is no clinical relevance. In other words, there has been no demonstration that people are helped through the use of these devices.

Therefore, in the opinion of this writer, the use of ozone for clinical indoor purposes is unwarranted.

Chapter 2
Humidifiers and Dehumidifiers

Humidifiers

If you wake up with a dry, scratchy throat, or your skin and scalp itch, then the air in your house may be too dry. Turning on the furnace in the winter, lighting a fire, or starting any other heating source will remove moisture from the air and can lead to one or more of these problems.

A humidifier can help, if you remember that humidifiers have potential problems of their own. If you have asthma, it may be just what the doctor ordered.

There are a number of things to consider when shopping for a humidifier to avoid getting into trouble. As a source of moisture, humidifiers can easily become contaminated with mold and bacterial growth; they must be easy to clean. Sometimes the manufacturer does not give the best recommendations regarding what to use to clean the device. It's possible to leave a residue that becomes problematic when you breathe it. Stick with something simple, such as vinegar or half a lemon.

If you buy an ultrasonic humidifier, beware of the following problems: Ultrasound causes the formation of micro-water droplets. If contaminating bacteria or mold are present, then the bacteria and mold particles are sonicated (ruptured and broken) into micro-fragments that are readily inhaled. Hard water and residual lime deposits can also be sonicated, and symptoms of lime inhalation can be similar to those of microbial inhalation, in my experience. So keep the unit clean and use distilled water. This is likely to be more expensive.

A humidistat on the machine is a device that displays the relative humidity (RH), but only the RH near the machine, because that is where it is attached. You are the best humidistat. Do not put too much faith in this gadget.

The wick type of humidifier is safest from the standpoint of microbial growth, although it is somewhat noisy.

Impeller types have fan blades that sling water into the air. They are easy to clean, but when contaminated can become a real problem. They require soft or distilled water, and this can cost more than the machine itself over a year's time.

Steam-mist types use a lot of energy. The heat will kill microorganisms, so filters aren't needed. However, they can still emit dead microbes when they become contaminated. It is important to understand that dead and live microbes both have allergenic properties.

Tabletop humidifiers should have a portable tank with handles or side grips for convenience, and a large enough capacity to humidify a medium to large-size room. Console models should have casters or wheels and a switch that shuts off the unit when the water tank is low or empty. Units of this size are touted to humidify an entire home and will often have a humidistat. In any case, buy a unit that opens wide for ease of cleaning (about once weekly).

Be conservative in your efforts to add moisture to your lives. Remember that dust mites are prolific when the RH gets above 65 percent.

Dehumidifiers

Dehumidifiers are similar to air-conditioning in that they remove moisture from the air. They are important in various areas of the home where excessive moisture may be present, such as bathrooms and basements.

Tens of millions of homes do not have air-conditioning, but require a device that can remove excessive moisture; other homes may be air-conditioned and still have a basement.

Frequently, basements have a high moisture content for various reasons and might require the use of a dehumidifier with a high capacity to remove moisture from the air. This is especially true when the RH is above 65 percent. The goal is to reach an RH below the 50 percent level. This will minimize the chances that mold growth will occur on the walls and contents of the area. The moisture must be drained. Many units will capture the water into a tray that may be emptied every day or twice a day. Alternatively, the dehu can exit the water directly into a floor drain or connect to a screw-on hose that leads to the floor drain.

When purchasing a dehu, look for the features that include a screw-on hose connection, return policy, and guarantee.

Combination dehumidifier/humidifiers that connect to the furnace are available.

Also, if you need one for another area of the home, shop wisely. (Please see the chapter on portable air purifiers).

Chapter 3

Air Filters

────────────

There are a wide variety of filters available for the central heating and cooling system of the home. These fall into several categories: passive electrostatic, electronic, active air filtration, and special filters.

For any central air filter to work to its highest capability, the air must flow through it for at least eight hours a day. A filter will not work if air and the particles (and gases) it contains do not come in contact with it.

Passive electrostatic filters are well marketed, but there is little evidence that their use causes a substantial reduction in the amount of house dust. Their operating principle is that they develop an electronic negative charge as air passes through their mesh. The principle is similar to the positively charged dust that is attracted to a negatively charged television screen. An advantage to the use of these filters is that they are reusable; people can save money by washing them off and replacing them back into the unit rather than buying more. They are also inexpensive. Finally, they can be charged without electricity passing through them (and generating ozone).

The primary disadvantage is that the passive electrostatic filter does not remove finer dust particles, the bulk of which constitute airborne particulates. The filter actually increases in efficiency as it becomes more loaded. They are inexpensive because they are rated by some as being in the low to low-moderate range of capability.

Electrically charged (electronic) filters require the construction of a special central unit to house them. An electrical charge is sent through the grate, attracting dust particles of virtually all sizes. The grate can be hosed off to free it from the dust load. Its greatest virtue is that it is highly efficient. Its disadvantages are that it is expensive to install and will produce ozone, a respiratory irritant. Older units do worse in this regard than the newer models, which are greatly improved.

If the reader is interested in investigating the purchase of a central air handling device, then I would suggest shopping around. (The reader must understand that virtually no proof has been presented that links the removal of particulates from the indoor air and improvement in health, despite numerous media reports to the contrary.)

Active air filtration filters are generally made of synthetic weave materials and are quite inexpensive. Some cost less than a dollar each. The see-through types are very inefficient and do little, if anything, to remove particles from the air. Similar to passive electrostatics, they improve in efficiency over time, once they get dirty and the pore size diminishes. At this point, clumps of dust may break off to enter the airstream.

Accordion weave or pleated filters are much better, and are readily available in most hardware stores. The 3M Company is reputed to make a good-quality pleated filter in the five to seven dollar range and it should filter much better than others that might sell for the same price or less.

Space Guard (Gard) is a company that must retrofit your unit to take in their large pleated filter. However, their filter has a reputation for being quite efficient, and the replacement filters are relatively inexpensive. They appear to be better than most alternative filtration processes in terms of filtration ability and convenience of filter replacement.

HEPA (high efficiency particulate air) filters have been state of the art for decades and are used in nuclear power plants and surgical rooms. A central unit must be created around the filter for it to operate. This is because the weave is so thick that it would block airflow if one tried to insert the HEPA into an average unit.

HEPA-like filters are almost universally available. Do not be confused by the words, as they do not filter at the capacity that the true HEPA does. However, their price range may be more acceptable.

Special filters are available online or from filter manufacturers in big cities. Frequently, requests are made for pleated filters that contain activated charcoal. (Try making coffee with whole beans versus finely ground powder.) In other words, the charcoal is much more efficient if ground to finer granules. These granules can be added to pleated filters for removal of particulates along with many volatile organic compounds.

One disadvantage of a carbon addition to filters is that, if they are overloaded, the saturated carbon will outgas the odor back into the room. One example is with the odors of paint. Consider carbon to be a temporary fix until the source of the odor can be identified and removed through fresh-air flushing of the home. Odors include those from painting, gluing, varnishing, polishing, and other household activities. A disadvantage is that the carbon must be discarded and cannot be recharged.

Zeolite rock is made from volcanic ash and is excellent at absorbing small-molecule odors such as ammonia and formaldehyde. For example, a tiny bag of zeolite placed in the refrigerator will absorb the odors of a large amount of pastrami. Zeolite is inexpensive and can be placed in the sun where the odors will evaporate. Unlike carbon filters, the material can be recycled.

Filters with three absorbents—carbon, zeolite, and potassium permanganate—are also available, for filtration of large and small molecule gases. These include ammonia, formaldehyde, perfumes, fragrances, varnishes, polishes, glues, and other respiratory irritants.

Chapter 4

Air-Handling Systems

Back in a 1989 report to Congress, the EPA stated that "sufficient evidence exists to conclude that indoor air pollution represents a major portion of the public's exposure to air pollution and may pose serious acute and chronic health risks."[2] The focus here is on office buildings, hospitals, and schools, but it is obvious that what they say can apply to homes.

Given that heating, ventilation, and air-conditioning (HVAC) equipment is in place, most professionals will agree that problems are rarely with the equipment itself. When air quality issues in buildings arise, then one should look at overloaded equipment and misused airspace. For example, air-conditioning drip pans that are maintained poorly, fill with debris, and do not drain properly permit the buildup of mold and bacteria and an overflow of the pan. Other examples include infrequent changing of HVAC filters, using the wrong filters for the system, placing fresh-air intakes downwind from exhaust vents, or placing ten people in a space meant for two.

Remember that air-conditioning in buildings or homes does not remove smells, it just dilutes them. This is because in commercial systems, there is usually a certain amount of fresh air that is let in at the unit itself at a recommended twenty cubic feet per minute per person. Frequently, the renovation process overloads the indoor air with the smells of adhesives, new carpeting, and paint without adequate warning to the building inhabitants. Many of us have experienced this gross lack of concern by building management at one time or another.

It is possible to obtain activated carbon filters that will remove indoor odors without impeding airflow. These are available through air filtration companies commonly listed in city telephone directories.

It is the responsibility of building management to advise building inhabitants to use commonsense ventilation. This means that those who are leasing the building and the management both share in the responsibility of maintaining clean air. And using a state-of-the-art air filtration system is no excuse for carelessness. One cannot buy a car with airbags, then drive recklessly and still expect to be safe!

Many experts advocate the prohibition of the introduction of chemicals into the HVAC system. This system includes the air ducts, except when required in an emergency or unusual situation. In that event, complete information should be provided to building occupants before any such action is undertaken. This avoids unnecessary health risks, complaints, and lawsuits.

There should not be an introduction of such additives as deodorizers, disinfectants, perfumes, scents, ozone, or other aromas into the HVAC system. These additions to the air encourage and contribute to the development of sick buildings and unhappy occupants.

Pine-scented products, and most particularly air fresheners used to mask troubling odors, can be debilitating for those already sick from indoor pollutants. They can be annoying and can interfere with worker efficiency.

We should strive to appreciate air without smell. We should also encourage the use of self-operating, ratcheted or sliding, transparent, silicon-derived ventilation systems—also known as windows.

Chapter 5

Portable Air Purifiers

Conventional thought has it that removal of particles from the air will provide for better health. This has never been proven. It is too difficult to set up credible tests that will prove or disprove this claim. All we can do is to determine that particles and gases have been removed, and then intuitively assert that there is great benefit to this event.

Most portable air purifiers will provide a prefilter for larger dust particles, a carbon filter for odors, and a high-efficiency HEPA filter for fine particles. Many of these units will run the carbon first as a prefilter. This is an incorrect arrangement. The micropores present in carbon particles will be blocked by dust in the air, ending the ability of the carbon to remove odors very quickly. Almost all experts agree that a prefilter should be the first filter to catch the dust and to screen out the larger particles.

The amount of carbon used in any unit is relatively small and should not be measured by its weight. The finer the carbon, the better it will absorb volatile organic compounds. However, be aware that at some point, every carbon filter will overload. Thus, the carbon may need to be changed more frequently than the manufacturer recommends. The number of weeks or months that you change the filter will depend on usage.

A word of caution: There are dozens, if not scores, of companies that make portable air purifiers. As is true for ozone-generating machines, there has never been a single published reproducible study in a reputable peer-reviewed scientific or medical journal that has shown a lessening of symptoms in the home when the units were used. That's a strong statement. Marginal studies were not sufficient to convince the medical community because they could not be duplicated and in a large percentage of cases, the data obtained from control groups could not be distinguished from those obtained from experimental groups. This is probably true of vacuum cleaners, as well.

Let's give an example. In a very simple experimental format, we have twenty people, ten who are allergic or asthmatic and ten who are not. Because 85 percent of asthma is allergic asthma, we run into our first problem—separating the two groups. Simply put, the parameters of a study are difficult to define. Even if we manage to have two separate groups, we need to adjust for age, sex, and other factors. The second problem then comes into play. Do we count the number of times each of ten people sneezes, or the number of times their eyes itch and water? Even if we have only one group of ten asthmatic people and we want to measure the number of asthma attacks that occur before, during and after our air purifier was used, we run into problems again. How severe are the attacks? How long do we run the air purifier and in what room(s) prior to measuring the number of attacks? If we put it in the person's bedroom, we can certainly measure the level of particle reduction, but not for the triggering of an attack from perfume, the smell of cooked onions, or for a trip to the store or to school. Thus, we cannot adequately *control* our experiment unless our subjects are kept in controlled housing with controlled foods.

Also, the knowledge that an air purifier is working for them could lessen the number and severity of symptoms. This is called the placebo effect. Therefore, we are back to a couple of study groups, some who know that their air purifier is working and some who are not told that the purifier they have been given doesn't have a HEPA filter or carbon.

Suffice it to say air purifiers are only part of the solution, not the answer to the problem. Maintaining a dust-free home is another part of the equation for reduction in allergen exposures.

There is no doubt that the air-purifier industry is huge. As with everything else, there is a right way and a wrong way to do things.

If you believe a unit will be helpful for you or your family, then I will present some parameters that will help you choose one that is right for you.

The ideal air purifier should have several qualities. Solid construction is one of them. Many people prefer a unit constructed of metal rather than plastic. This tends to make them more durable, which can be important when children are present in the home. It also tends to make them heavier; not a problem for most people.

Another factor is sound. The purifier should have several settings for speed and be relatively quiet when in operation. The consumer will soon get used to the sound of the motor, however, and it will tend to block out background noise. This turns out to be a plus in the opinion of many users.

The ideal air purifier should have lots of carbon. It is better yet to have additives such as zeolite and potassium permanganate. Zeolite is crushed volcanic rock that is very good at absorbing hydrogen sulfide (from sewer gases) and small molecule ammonia-type smells (pastrami in the refrigerator). The carbon takes care of the rest of the odors, including glues, perfumes, and paints. An air purifier should have a long-lasting warranty and a return policy. Like humidifiers, larger units should have wheels.

It is important for the consumer to take notes while shopping for an air purifier. Claims are easy to make; true workability is a different matter. Compare the efficiency of one brand with another, but don't expect to filter the entire home with a portable air purifier.

Be advised that standard air cleaners will not remove formaldehyde from the air to any significant extent because carbon-base filtration does not work in this regard. If you do buy an air purifier, get a unit that can go into the master bedroom or child's room. Make sure it is rugged and has a good guarantee. Factor in the cost of replacement filters when you purchase the unit.

Beware of claims that say a particular brand will make you feel better. That is false advertising and the federal government frowns on it. So does common sense. If you hear of such a claim, ask to see evidence that it works, not testimonials.

At best, a portable air cleaner will remove airborne dust nearest the unit. It will not remove the dust on your bed covering, under the bed, in the carpets, on the sofa, on windowsills, or on the TV screen. You will have to do that part.

Chapter 6

Vacuum Cleaners

You think you need a new vacuum cleaner, but you don't know what to buy. Before you get too involved in the shopping process, take another look at your old unit. If it is a canister and the only problem is that it leaks dust into the air, try using duct tape to wrap the area where the hose fits into the canister. If it is an upright, then you might want to call around for higher-quality bags. If you have made up your mind to get a new vacuum cleaner, first review some basics.

Be wary of too many gadgets. Most people require something that is versatile, is easy to roll around, and has a good strong suction. As always, price is only one factor in choosing a new product and is not always a good way to compare different models.

Over the past few years, *Consumer Reports Buying Guides* have suggested that the middle range of prices will provide a good vacuum cleaner for the average person and the average need. At that price one can get a unit with a cleaning path of some fourteen inches, good-quality bags, and a wider range of tools than less expensive models.

Uprights generally work better on carpets, but many also perform well on bare flooring. If you need a lot of attachments for specialized cleaning jobs, such as underneath beds and furniture, and you have a lot of bare flooring, then a canister will probably work best for you. After inspecting under beds, most people can testify that cleaning there is an important chore.

Canisters are also quieter than uprights and do a better job on carpeted stairs.

Cord length is a consideration. The average length is twenty to thirty feet and many canisters have retractable cords, although uprights are easier to store. Some upright units feature an upper cord-wrap device that swivels down to release the cord immediately, rather than requiring the user to unwind it coil-by-coil.

If you opt for a unit with no bags, remember that you will still have to empty the container. Preferably, this should be done outdoors.

Unless you decide to buy a vacuum cleaner with a *full-dirt* indicator, you will have to change your bag on a regular basis. This may not be what you want, as it is just one more thing that can go wrong. It is better for the user to be in control and remember that when a bag gets full, the suction power is reduced.

HEPA filtration sounds good, but there is no way to tell if the unit is constructed well enough to do what it is supposed to do. In fact, *Science News* reported that HEPA vacuum cleaners are no better at protecting against dust mites than standard models. The report also states that both HEPA and non-HEPA units can actually increase an individual's exposure to particles containing cat antigens.[7]

Be aware that if you have small children in the home, they will often leave small objects on the floor. This is important because the blower fan in most vacuums is made of plastic, and it is this fan which drives the dirt into the bag. It is also breakable. Some units are constructed in such a manner that the dirt is filtered through the bag before reaching the fan. Hence, no breakage.

A suction control is present on canisters. It is used for doing draperies and specialized objects.

Uprights frequently allow for increased suction by lowering or raising the unit from the carpet or floor surface. This is fine, but try to choose a model with large rear wheels to make the pushing easier.

Here's an important point: suction power is only one factor involved in pulling up dirt. In a word, don't get enamored with the sales pitch that focuses on this factor. Filtration, variable distance from the floor, cost, return policy, warrantee, and other factors should factor into the equation. A badly designed unit can offset suction power, and many less expensive units can clean just as well as the most expensive models out there.

Another important point: successful cleaning is shared between the cleaner and the 'cleanee'. The carpeting industry tells us that slow cross-wise vacuuming is a lot more important than fast back-and-forth motion. Why? Because the first removes dirt most effectively, and the second scatters it into the air, which provides ample dust for the user to inhale.

Make sure you purchase an attachment that can get those areas between the carpeting and the base of the walls, between the sofa cushions, between the refrigerator and counter and walls, between the box spring and the frame, and between the number and type of crevices that present themselves in every home.

You may need some sort of hand attachment to get the surface of the sofa and armchairs, where an incredible amount of dust accumulates in a short period of time.

Plan first. Then decide how much you want to spend and what features you require according to the needs of your household. Make sure that quality bags are available for the unit and that you can afford to buy them on a regular basis.

Chapter 7

Refrigerators

If you want to lessen the load on your lungs and your health in general, then clean the refrigerator. It may be the most disease-transmitting area of the entire home.

There are ten or more areas of the fridge that can catch you by surprise, and you need to check them on a regular basis. These include handles and outside surfaces, the refrigerator top, the door seals and paint, the vegetable and meat drawers, the food itself, the drain hole, the drip pan, the floor beneath the unit, the fan, and the wall behind it. If you have a family, odds are that you've got some work ahead of you.

The rubber seals around the doors of the refrigerator and freezer frequently have food particles that have accumulated over the years. These frequently support the growth of green-black mold. Allergenic *Cladosporium* (*Hormodendrum*) is the common mold here. Its spores are liberated into the air space when the door is opened. Fortunately, the number liberated is low. The bad news is that this mold will also degrade the integrity of the seal over time.

The grooves of the seal are easy to clean. Use a damp soapy washcloth or cotton swab to clean them. The mold will come off readily.

In addition, this mold growth can occur on the paint, where the doors meet the body of the unit. A warm soapy washcloth will remove this scum. If you use a sponge, microwave it for sixty seconds after use to sterilize it.

Pull out the vegetable and meat drawers. Take out the food

and clean out any pools of water within and beneath the drawers. This water is usually contaminated by microbes, including a wide variety of bacteria that have adapted to colder temperatures. Examine the food itself and discard soggy and decayed vegetables, fruits, breads, and other suspect items.

If you are thinking about eating the moldy cheese to get free antibiotics, forget it. Although the green mold that contaminates cheese, bread, and fruits is usually *Penicillium*, you may inhale allergenic spores in the process. These spores will be liberated into the kitchen and home, and while they may not grow elsewhere as a result of this liberation, they can certainly add to the allergen load of the airspace.

Open old jam jars and check for mold growth on the surface of the product and where the lid connects to the jar. If the jam has an alcohol smell, discard it. Yeasts, which are a subdivision of molds, are at work here. If the pancake syrup has something growing on the top of it, discard it.

When food gets low, it might be a good idea to empty the entire refrigerator and clean it completely with a solution of baking soda—one-half cup in a gallon of warm water. When you put the food back in, you may want to include a small dish of baking soda to absorb odors.

Make sure the hole to the drain pan is open and unclogged. A hole for runoff of water condensation is present in older units. This water goes to the drain pan underneath the refrigerator. In older units this hole is located inside and at the back between the vegetable drawers. A pool of standing water in that spot is a sure indication that the hole is plugged. Bacteria will be growing in this water. Soak up the excess water with paper towels and discard them. Usually the hole can be opened with a wire.

Pull out the grate at the bottom of the unit and take a look underneath. Most under-fridge areas have dust-balls along with fine dirt, pollen, spores, and allergenic insects and their parts. You may find some surprises in the form of an object that you once lost. Warm air from the motor causes the finer particles to become airborne. That's a lot of exposure considering the number of family hours that are spent in and near the kitchen. The unit will have to be unplugged and pulled out, and the floor carefully swept and then damp-mopped.

While the unit is out, be sure to carefully clean the area around the fan. This cleaning will help avoid expensive repair bills, as the fan will cease operation once it becomes clogged with dirt. When the fan stops, so does the refrigeration.

Once the refrigerator is pulled out, don't forget to wipe down the walls beside and behind it. And be careful not to injure the cooling coils while you pull out and return the unit. Gently clean the coils while you are at it.

Next, while the bottom grate is off, pull out and wash the drain pan that is present in most older refrigerators. You will need to pull out the grate at the bottom of the unit and, unfortunately, get down on your hands and knees to locate the drain pan.

As everyone knows, the top of the fridge accumulates a lot of dust and grease because it is above eye level and is frequently located near the stove. This area should be washed with a damp warm washcloth or sponge and dishwashing detergent. Then wash out the sponge and put it in the microwave on high for sixty seconds to sterilize it. You should be thoroughly wetting and microwaving the sponge daily, in any case.

Finally, don't neglect to wipe the handle and front and sides of the unit after putting back in place. (Use a 1:10 dilution of chlorine bleach.) This is one of the dirtiest and most contaminated areas of the entire home, as everyone touches the front and sides of fridge (and the vegetable drawers). (Please refer to the chapter on viruses and bacteria in the home.)

Temperature control settings in the refrigerator (and freezer) are important tools for keeping food fresh, cold, and usable. You may need to turn down the settings if there is little food present and turn it up when there is more. Remember that cold air travels downward so the bottom shelf will tend to be cooler than the others. Also, never put hot foods or liquids into the unit since this will raise the temperature for an extended period and may cause the spoiling of food that is already present, including dairy products, fruits, vegetables, and meats. Bacteria that cause serious food poisoning may reproduce rapidly in the warmer conditions. These would include *E. coli*, *Salmonella*, and *Staphylococcus*.

Chapter 8
Central Air-Conditioning Systems

Many people believe that a better filter will remove bad smells from the home. This is true, but only to an extent, as virtually all the filters in use are oriented toward the removal of particulates. This means that gases will be filtered when they are attached to dust-like particles. Most of the gas molecules, however, are mixed in with the air. These are the main source of the odor and will pass through even the best paper or fiber filters.

If odors are your concern, either remove the source or go to carbon or zeolite filters. In any case, whether you have air-conditioning or not, the ideal home should be completely aired on a regular basis. The time frames for airing can range from as often as once or twice monthly, to whenever it can be accomplished, to virtually never, depending on your indoor problem and your local climate. In addition, heavily polluted areas may dictate that the air is better indoors than outdoors almost all the time.

Air-conditioning units in commercial buildings have a certain percentage of fresh air—20 percent—that is pulled into the building, as dictated by ASHRAE. This air is mixed with the inside air, cooled, and filtered. Sometimes, even this is not enough to dilute smells, such as those that originate from the adhesives used to glue down new commercial carpeting.

In the home, all of the interior air is recirculated with no fresh air. The exceptions to this are what you let in by entry and exit through the doors, the occasional opening of windows, or leakage. Odors are mixed and spread throughout the home to be absorbed into soft furnishings, wallboard, wallpaper, and clothes that are hanging in the closet.

When air is recirculated in an AC home, it travels through the duct system. Because a significant number of home duct systems have leaks, there will be some air exchange with the outside. This is unwanted from an energy standpoint. A great deal of heating or cooling energy will be lost.

A leaky air duct system means that a pressure differential will pull particles into the home. While a lot of the particles will be filtered, contaminants such as mold (from outdoors, or from a contaminated attic) or automotive gases will enter the home before they can be filtered.

Apartments offer special circumstances that pertain to air-conditioning and odors. This is because air conditioning creates positive pressure relative to other connecting units that have air conditioning which might not be in use. The unit(s) that utilize air conditioning will 'push' air through leaks in the electrical outlets, recessed lighting fixtures, and open cavities present where piping and wiring enter the walls (washer and dryer hookups and under-sink areas). Obviously, if a door or window is open to any extent, smoke and cooking odors will exit one unit only to enter others.

Independent of air-conditioning, normal airflow in a given room will vary depending on the time of the day. In the morning, as the sun warms the roof, the airflow will travel in a clockwise direction around a given room to carry dust along with it. In the evening, the airflow will occur in the opposite direction.

The air conditioning system will have a condensate line within a wall cavity that drains water from the pan to the sewer system or outdoors along side the home. This line can run through the wall cavity in the bathroom/bedroom or in the dining room, or elsewhere. Occasionally, the line may become clogged and can cause serious problems due to water leakage inside the home. It might be a good idea to find out where your condensate line is located, then inspect that area when you go on your occasional walk-through of the home.

If the line becomes clogged, water may accumulate over a period of days to years before it becomes evident because the leakage may be slow and the evaporation rate slow as well. However, realize that if the leakage is determined to have occurred over a longer period, your homeowner insurance policy will probably not pay on the repairs, and in addition, they will not pay for mold removal and testing. Insurance is tuned to sudden water loss and not loss over time (which you should have discovered on your own).

Chapter 9

Window Air Conditioners

The most common types of mold species that are blown into a home from the window air conditioner are members of the *Penicillium* and *Aspergillus* groups.

The common green bread and cheese mold can grow just as fast inside the refrigerator as outside of it. These are common bad-guy molds. They grow at a wide range of temperatures, in a wide range of humidities and utilize outdoor leaves and grasses, indoor foods and construction materials as a food source, including the components of indoor dust. Their spores are extremely small and extremely numerous. This means they can enter the deeper lungs (especially the *Aspergillus* group) to cause problems in allergic, asthmatic, and immunocompromised patients. It has been documented many times over that this last group of people can actually have *Aspergillus* growing inside of the lungs. These molds love a dirty and moist filter because they love dirt. Keep that filter clean.

The evaporator coil is inside the air-conditioning unit. It's the cold part of the unit. The air conditioning removes moisture from the air. During the rainy season, the air is very humid, so a lot more moisture will be removed. This moisture forms on the coil and can harbor mold growth, similar to AC coils in a car.

After water condenses on the evaporator coil, it drips into the drain pan. The pan has a hole in it so the water can drain out. Sometimes debris can clog the hole and water will accumulate in the pan, similar to the interior of an older refrigerator. Microbial growth will occur in this mess, and so will its accompanying smell.

The window unit should be level; otherwise moisture can run into the home. This is another problem that will occur if the drain pan is clogged.

Chapter 10

Evaporative Coolers

Tens of millions of people in the Southwestern United States and desert areas of the Pacific Northwest use evaporative coolers (ECs) in homes, businesses, and schools. Many of those EC users suffer from allergies and believe that air-conditioning is better for their health.

In truth, the jury is still out on this issue. Many people who find fault with ECs often use them improperly. The EC is so widely abused, it's a wonder that more people don't become sick from its use. Alternatively, maybe you are ill but don't know that the cooler caused your problem.

The EC, also known as a swamp cooler, consists of a large box that is vented on three or four sides, depending on whether it is mounted to the side of a building or on the roof. Inside the removable sides are large pads made of aspen fibers or cellulose. The pads are continually wet from a sump located at the bottom of the box and a network of tubes that feeds the water into the pads. A generator drives a large squirrel cage inside the unit to send the moistened air into the building. When windows are opened slightly, excellent indoor cooling is maintained, unless the humidity outdoors becomes elevated.

Over months of use, if it isn't cleaned on a regular basis, the EC can load up with lime, bacteria, mold, leaves, and mosquitoes. There are reports of schools that turned on the cooler at the beginning of the season, sending live mosquitoes into the classrooms at high speed, frightening teachers and students.

It is a safe bet that many of the same people who complain

about indoor illness from the EC haven't cleaned it in a long time.

When properly used and maintained, the EC will blow particles of indoor dust, dirt, and accumulated allergens out the windows and provide good cooling at the same time. Proper use of the EC calls for getting the pads very wet before turning on the blower. This keeps hot dry flakes of lime from blowing into the home when you first turn it on. When inhaled, lime dust can mimic allergies and may precipitate an asthma attack.

Here are a couple of hints for proper use of the EC: Close or decrease the registers in the rooms you are not using. This will lend more force to the other vents. You may be able to use a lower-power setting as a result and save money. Redirect any register that blows air right on your head, such as when you are standing in the kitchen or seated in an armchair. This factor alone can tend to aggravate allergies and asthma due to excessive cooling. Even otherwise normal folks can get what is called a 'fan hangover' if this is allowed to occur. If you have a fan pointed at your head while you are sleeping you can wake up feeling very groggy, stuffy, and wiped out. This is similar to the effect caused by a table fan directed toward your head.

A number of factors affect how open a window should be for optimal cooling with an EC: size of the home and the cooler, whether the unit is on high or low, how many windows are open, and how many registers are closed. Generally, windows are open three to six inches for maximum cooling effect because the cool moist air must exit somewhere. If you hear a whistling sound, then you need to close or open a window more—the noise means air is rushing past the frame. Doors may also be opened.

If a window is open too much, there will not be enough

positive pressure in the home, and particles from the outside will enter the indoor environment, especially during breeze conditions. If a window is not open at all, then there will be very little cooling and the level of allergenic particles in the home will increase, along with the relative humidity. Once that happens, mold (usually *Penicillium*) will begin to grow on leather clothing such as hats, shoes, and belts inside of tightly packed closets, and it will quickly spread to contaminate the entire home.

The evaporative cooler has two big problems: microbes and lime. The water reservoir in the cooler usually contains a great deal of dirt, leaves, bugs, and nutrients to support a large population of microbial life., The water can harbor millions of bacteria per milliliter, enough to sour milk within a few hours if they are the right kind.[8]

Some of the cooler-water bacteria are potentially harmful and are certainly capable of causing respiratory irritation and infections, especially in the elderly and debilitated. Infections from coolers are more likely to occur when we feel rundown or have some other underlying infection. Just two of the diseases associated with evaporative coolers are humidifier fever and hypersensitivity pneumonitis. You don't have to be allergic to get these.

As stated above, mold becomes an important problem as well. Two of the most dangerous mold types that commonly inhabit the cooler are *Aspergillus* and *Fusarium*.[9] These allergenic molds are transmitted into the home.

The color of the water in the cooler reservoir cannot be considered a clue as to its relative cleanliness regarding microbes. It can go either way.

The accumulation of lime prevents the pads from absorbing water and evaporating it as water vapor. This cancels out the cooling effect by as many as three to five degrees Fahrenheit, in my experience, and also allows for the entry of free water droplets into the home rather than water vapor. The droplets can form on any surface, including the refrigerator or areas around the register itself. Usually, the dark green allergenic mold *Cladosporium* inhabits this ecological niche.

The cooler needs to be serviced about every eight to ten weeks. Scrub out the lime, change the pads, and service the belts if necessary. It should be serviced more frequently if there is a lot of blowing dust to contaminate it. After this period of time, microbial growth becomes significant. Only servicing the cooler at the start of the summer means that you will be at risk, and you'll also have lousy cooling as time goes on.

While there are a number of considerations to take into account when operating the humidifying device known as the evaporative cooler, it is an effective and inexpensive method to cool the air of a home or school. When the airflow is balanced, it can offer effective cooling to the building's inhabitants.

Endnotes

1. EPA. 2009. www.epa.gov/ozone.

2. EPA. 2008. Ozone generators that are sold as air cleaners. *Indoor Air Quality*. Dec. www.epa.gov/iaq/pubs/ozonen.html.

3. Federal Information and News Dispatch. 2009. Research Finds New Cause of Ozone Wheezing and Potential Treatments. *National Institutes of Health Documents*. Feb.

4. American Society for Heating, Refrigeration & Air Conditioning Engineers. 1989. *Fundamentals Handbook*. Pg 12. www.ashrae.org

5. Illinois Department of Public Health. 2009. *Ozone. Environmental Health Fact Sheet*. Feb. www.idph.state.il.us/envhealth/factsheets/ozone.htm

6. Nathanson, T. 1998 An Assessment of Ozone Generators. *Building Air Quality*. http://iaqconsultant.com/9.htm

7. University of Manchester. 2006. High Efficiency Vacuum Cleaners no Better at Protecting Against Dust Mites. *Science Daily*. Feb.

8. Sneller, M.R. and J.L. Pinnas, M.D. 1987.Comparison of airborne fungi in evaporative cooled and air conditioned homes. *Ann. Allergy* 59:317.

9. Ibid.

Section 9

Home Maintenance

Regardless of whether you live in a small or large house, or old or new home, or whether you live in an apartment, there are numerous ways to protect it from the outdoor climate while gaining energy efficiency and cleaner air at the same time. The tradeoff is a tighter dwelling with less fresh air to dilute out the toxic byproducts of normal living. The bad news is that these pollutants will add up to take time off our lives and keep us less healthy while that is occurring.

There is a basic rule that says: Whatever happens outdoors also happens indoors, but to a lesser extent and with a time delay. This rule applies to barometric pressure, dust particles, pollen, mold, and a variety of gases and particulates.

There are a number of research papers that demonstrate how PM10 particles enter the home from the outdoors. The degree that they enter depends on whether it is day or night (more enter during the day) and the amount of leakage in the home.[1,2,3] (Please refer to the chapter on Household Dust.)

Therefore, it behooves us to use less toxic cleaning and other household products for our daily indoor lives. This applies when the outdoor weather does not permit us to ventilate sufficiently and becomes particularly important for the home bound elderly, infants, or those who just cannot get outdoors for whatever reason. (Please see the section on Safe Household Cleaning.)

Chapter 1

Air Leaks

This segment refers to air leakage into our home. This leakage is basically related to energy inefficiency, but, depending on the home, can also relate to the entry of outdoor pollen and mold allergens.

There are a number of areas where outdoor air can enter a home: leaky windows and under doors; leaking air ducts; entry from the basement or attic; or use of the fireplace. All of these can be facilitated if the bathroom or kitchen fan is on to bring about negative pressure within the home.

Many people want a little leakage for the fresh air exchange. This is a good thing, especially if the indoor air needs to be diluted because of the use of an excess of fragrance products. This fresh air entry must be balanced with energy efficiency.

If you see spider webs in the corners of your windows, this is a sign that air leakage is occurring here. Spiders set up their webs next to openings where smaller creatures can enter.

When the damper is left open, the chimney is another source of leakage.

Plumbing fixtures have rings set against the walls. If the rings are not set tightly, then air from the inner wall spaces can enter or exit the home. This includes plumbing under sinks, bathtubs, and shower pipes that go into the wall.

It is common to find poorly sealed ductwork fittings off the main duct trunk. You may be able to determine this if you remove a register and, with the help of a flashlight, see if there is a tight fit of duct against the wall or a good fit between duct seams.

Poorly fitting registers are common in new homes. Air can be lost to wall cavities in this case.

Sometimes the tape that holds the ducting to the air conditioner and heater can become worn and permit the entry of outside, attic, crawl-space, or garage air into the home. What happens here is that air flows through a duct, creating a pressure differential relative to the air just at the inner walls of the duct. So, the airflow is positive, the walls are negative, and the outside air becomes relatively positive. Air is pulled into the duct to flow with the airstream.

Recessed lights and electrical fixtures may leak debris from the above-ceiling space when negative pressure is created within the home, if the fit is not tight.

Check the inside of your medicine cabinet. If it has metal brackets for the glass shelves, then these will open into the walls. This is a source of minor air leakage into the inner walls of the home.

Recessed sliding wooden doors may have huge leaks into the inner wall spaces. Fixing the problem here may be expensive.

If mold contamination exists within the framing of a wooden home, it is not hard to see the many ways that spores, or at least musty odors, can enter the home proper. When there is positive pressure within the home this is not a problem. When there is negative pressure, then odors will enter the reduced air pressure that is created, similar to outdoor breezes that move into an area of low pressure.

Air pressure changes are a common occurrence within homes for a variety of reasons.

Usually, the worst area for air system leakage is the return air system—that is, just before the air handler. Remove the return air register and take a good look behind it. You will probably see dirt, holes in the wall, lots of dust, evidence of insects and rodents, and construction materials. These all affect your breathing. The area should be cleaned out and damp-mopped, if this is the case. Don't forget to check the load and fit of the filter.

If there is a leak in the supply side of the system—that is, from the air handler to the interior space—this can be a serious problem. The result is negative pressure inside the home and the following pollutants can be drawn inside: radon gas, formaldehyde, pesticides, car exhaust from the garage, household cleaners, mold, and volatile organic compounds from several sources.

Negative pressure can occur under a number of other circumstances as well. For example, suppose you maintain the bedroom as a clean room and the door is closed. If there is no air supply register in the room or the register is closed, then negative pressure in the room can occur. This causes air to be pulled in from other rooms, and the clean room is no longer clean.

You can frequently tell which way air is flowing in a room by looking at the bottom of the door. You may see a strip of dirt along one side of the door. Or, you may see this strip of dirt in the carpet beneath the door as air passes under it. More dirt is present on the entry side.

The closet that houses the water heater should be treated as an outside closet and tightly sealed. Weather stripping will help here (as well as around windows). Roof vents in the closet serve to relieve excess gas that is generated, if the unit is gas powered. When the closet is inside the house, loosely fitting doors mean conditioned air will pass through the ill-fitting door and exit the roof vent.

A home can be checked by an infiltrometer, a computerized device that determines the location of leakages within a home and the extent of the leakages. Under normal circumstances, a 1,500-square-foot home should have about 1.2 square feet of total leakage area. On average, this leakage will exchange all the air in such a home with outside air at the recommended rate of eight to ten times each day.

Some of the duct leakages may be fixed by removing the registers and sealing any open space that exists between the duct and the wall.

Chapter 2
Air Duct Cleaning

Air duct cleaning (also known as HVAC remediation) is over a billion dollars strong in the United States. There is enough business in many communities for a dozen duct-cleaning companies. Many owners of such companies have engineering degrees and have a good understanding of the entire air-handling system. *In other cases, hired help leaves a lot to be desired in terms of their advice to the customer and knowledge about their profession.*

Each home is different. The age and general health of the furnace, lifestyles of the occupants, air conditioner, evaporative cooler, age of the air ducts, and style of the ducts (e.g., galvanized metal sheeting versus flex duct) can all vary. Homes are of different sizes and shapes. Some homes are located in dustier or more humid locations and need more frequent cleaning. While duct cleaning is not the cure-all, it does have its place in maintaining the overall health of the home. Unfortunately, it is extremely difficult to measure its effect on the home occupant scientifically, or with any degree of accuracy.

In a high percentage of homes, air ducts have a leakage problem. They can pull in particulates, gases, and allergens from the attic or the out-of-doors. When ducts leak, heating and cooling in the home is uneven. This can result in microbial contamination of the ducts and increase your power usage. If you are going to have your ducts cleaned, you should also ask about having them pressure-checked for leaks.

Who needs to have the ducts cleaned? Those who live in new homes with residual construction material, older homes that have not had their ducts cleaned, homes that have had a small fire or chemical spill (including extensive painting), homes with a rusty furnace, homes with a previous water leak beneath the air-handling plenum, homes that have been occupied by a cat or a smoker, or homes that have gone a few years without a cleaning.

Everyone should have their ducts pressure-checked for leaks, as leaky ducts are extremely common whether the home is new or old, and the amount of leakage can be astounding. In some cases it can be the equivalent of a hole several inches in height running across the living room wall.

What is the average amount of dust removed from the typical air duct? In terms of three-pound coffee cans, it ranges from between half a can to fifteen cans, with the average around two or three.

The registers (vents) should be disinfected periodically. There is some debate as to whether the ducts themselves need to be disinfected. Evaporative coolers deposit more grit in the ducts than air-conditioning systems. This is understandable. They contribute a lot of water vapor, which can condense onto the paint of the registers (vents) and walls immediately around and above the registers, providing a damp surface for microbial growth to occur. Typically, this growth consists of the allergenic mold known as *Cladosporium.* This mold loves to grow in air duct systems and wet paint.

Excess moisture leads to mold contamination in central air-handling systems. This occurs due to a number of reasons: The central humidifier is improperly installed. An air conditioning system is too small for the cubic footage that it has to serve. The cooling coils are dirty. There is poor moisture drainage from the drip pan, usually due to blockage. If this is the case, mold growth on the sheetrock or gypsum board should be evident.

(Note: NADCA, or the North American Duct Cleaners Association,[4] recommends against the addition of any agent to the air duct system unless extreme circumstances exist. In other words, industry standards suggest not using chemicals to clean either the air ducts or the return of the air conveyance system unless there has been smoke or mold damage. Then, the only products permissible to use should be labeled and EPA registered for that specific use.)

What should the consumer be concerned with when looking for a reputable air duct cleaning company? First, find out if they are licensed, bonded, and insured. This allows the consumer some recourse if the business does not live up to its promises. And as always, shop around and compare prices and services.

Two products include Oxine, which is used for HVAC cleaning, and Alka-Brite, used for cleaning coils.

Note that flex ducting in newer homes cannot be effectively cleaned for mold contamination. You should replace it instead of using an encapsulating agent.

Treat the air-handling system of the home like you would treat yourself or your car. Subject it to a quarterly inspection to ascertain the repairs that need to be accomplished.

Chapter 3

Nontoxic Building
and Repair Materials

There is an ongoing interest in the relative toxicity of construction materials, and numerous and excellent books have been
written on the subject.[5,6,7] This short piece is meant to introduce
the reader to a few of the most common construction and repair materials and their irritant or nontoxic nature.

While carpeting is not part of a house's building materials,
it is attached to the home, and in real estate terms, that quali-
fies it as part of the structure. The carpet has been discussed in
other areas of this volume.

Concrete foundations. These are usually acceptable after
curing unless they are treated with formaldehyde, petroleum
oils, or detergents. Slabs may contain pesticides that outgas
into the carpeting and the home when cracks develop. Check
with your builder regarding the details of the materials he is
using. He may buy in bulk and may not know the answer. In
this case the supplier must be contacted.

Masonry foundations. These are more permeable than concrete to moisture and radon gas.

Steel frames. These may be coated with oily residue from
the factory. The residue can be removed with detergent.

Glues. Normally used are white glue and yellow glue containing acrylics, casein, and/or vinyl acetate, but no petroleum
solvents. Wallpaper glue usually has a starch base, which is

okay, but some commercial glues contain mold retardants and pesticides to prevent their degradation by insects.

Wall tile adhesive. Be aware that these products usually contain toluene, benzene, and naphtha—three carcinogens. Once covered and sealed by tile and grout, its presence is not a problem. Use plenty of fresh air when applying it.

Floor tile adhesive. Please see the chapter on floor coverings.

Silicone sealants. The clear variety is best once it dries. Linseed oil putty is also widely acceptable. Butyl rubber and acrylic sealants are the most unacceptable.

Cabinets. The best units have a metal frame and doors; the worst are made of hardwood veneered "cabinet stock" along with standard particle board and vinyl "imitation wood" panels, which outgas petrochemical derivatives and formaldehyde.

Pipes. Copper pipes with mechanical joints are better than copper pipes with lead-soldered joints; galvanized steel is lined with zinc, which can enter the water supply upon reaction with chlorine; PVC contains vinyl chloride, a human carcinogen; polybutylene tubing will spring leaks, which will lead to water damage, subsequent mold growth, and expensive repair bills.

Chapter 4

Floor Coverings

There are a lot of choices when it comes to floor coverings, and different people have different needs. What we all have to be concerned with is this: which ones are the easiest to maintain for people who care about their respiratory health? Let's look at the pros and cons of these choices.

Many believe that the safest area rugs are made from untreated natural fibers, as opposed to pretreated or spray-on stain-resistant chemicals. This is only partly true. Some may contain chemical dyes, residual pesticide, and mothproofing. Cotton is treated while still on the plant to reduce the infestation of boll weevils, mites, and budworms still present in many areas of the country. (These and other insects destroy cotton boll, consume the seeds and flowers of the plant, and require a variety of pesticides to reduce their incidence.)

The wool is treated prior to shearing of the sheep. The animal is immersed in a chemical solution of pesticides to kill pests such as mites and lice.[8]

Pesticides, such as malathion and permethrin, are used in sheep wool production and are more of a threat to soil, groundwater, and handlers than they are to the end user of the wool. This is because processing of the wool will remove virtually all the pesticides.[9,10]

Lanolin is a byproduct of production of sheep wool shearing where it is present in the wool itself and in the sebaceous glands of the animal. It is readily absorbed in the human skin for moisturizing purposes and will not become rancid upon standing.

Many types of floor coverings may be a problem during installation. These include glued-down carpeting, soft vinyl tile, self-adhesive tile, simulated wood flooring, and foam rubber carpet pads. The volatile organic compounds (VOCs) emitted from the glues and textiles are respiratory and eye irritants. Fortunately, under normal conditions when fresh air is supplied, these VOCs will dissipate within hours to days.

Carpet is easiest to clean when it is of the commercial variety and low pile. When wet, it will be free from mold growth if it is made of nylon, rayon, or other synthetics. The pad can grow mold if wet because it is frequently a cellulose-base product, and mold is hard-wired to digest cellulose. Also, the paper/cellulose strip that is used on the underside of carpets to join together two pieces is probably the first place that mold will attack once a carpet gets wet.

Synthetic carpets are stain resistant. The more shallow weave is easier to vacuum and will hold less dirt, pesticides, and other contaminants. A spill that occurs on a carpet will spread throughout its base. The fibers will wick it up to cause surface staining in many cases, even after you sop up the surface wetness. Once a spill occurs or a stain-causing agent has soaked into a carpet, several treatments may be required to remove the causative agent.

If you're going to buy a new carpet, be aware that some people react to nylon when they come into contact with it.

After installation, new carpets should be vacuumed very slowly to pull up loose fibers that can otherwise be airborne. Once airborne, the fibers will be inhaled or burned off in the heater to create toxic gases and particles, although they will probably not be inhaled to any meaningful degree.

Astroturf is made of polypropylene, usually with a vinyl or rubber backing. It is relatively safe, but obviously it has limited uses indoors. Indoor/Outdoor is similar. It can be used in play-rooms or in the patio; it shows dirt readily. It is fairly easy to clean, but does not wear evenly. Frequently, areas of tracking become readily apparent.

Vinyl tile squares will go over wood or concrete nicely. There are advantages here. Damaged tiles can be replaced and cracks in the slab can be covered. An endless variety of patterns are available. You can install it yourself. It keeps down humidity in the home during the rainy season, or otherwise wet climates, by acting as a vapor barrier on the top of the concrete slab. This is more important than it might seem at first glance. Cracks in the slab will permit under-home pesticides to migrate upward into the living area under certain conditions.

If you decide to use vinyl tile, you will still need to deal with the glue. Because the tile will be laid over the glue (which may be at the base of the tile or sold separately), the off-gassing from the glue will be minimal. Fresh air will help here.

Keep the patterns simple. The more complicated the design, the more grooves will be in the tile and the more dirt will be retained. Also, it will still have to be waxed occasionally. Make sure you have several squares and some glue left over for replacement purposes later.

After installation, mop the new floor with warm soapy water to remove any excess of new product chemicals. These are volatile; that is, they can be airborne readily.

Used beneath vinyl flooring, the mastic has a high predilection for mold growth (especially *Stachybotrys*), once the underside becomes saturated from water. Under normal conditions of dampness, it poses no problems regarding contamination. Avoid cleaning the vinyl with any commercial product that contains petroleum distillates, as these products outgas significantly to contaminate the air.

The basic idea is that you want flooring that is very easily applied, retains and shows as little dirt as possible, and can outgas very quickly during and after installation.

Concrete is one possibility. There are even artists who can paint marvelous scenes on your concrete flooring. But concrete can be cold, and it cracks, allowing under-the-home pesticides to come indoors.

Ceramic tile looks good, can be damp-mopped, and is easily swept. Broken pieces can be replaced or used in combination with other types of floor covering such as low-pile Berber carpeting. Ceramic tile is a great nontoxic, low-dust floor covering.

Saltillo tile is similar to ceramic tile, but requires waxing and fairly regular care. The level of volatile chemical irritants in the home can be seriously elevated from their care products unless you carefully select them.

Linoleum is the grandfather of vinyl. It is made of cork, wood, and mineral chips bound by hardened linseed oil on a canvas backing. It grows brittle over time and is less stain resistant and chemical resistant than modern vinyl. Both can be cleaned with half a cup of white vinegar in a gallon of warm water.

Area carpets have their purpose. There is no way to know the pesticide content in cotton fibers. You may want to choose a synthetic weave unless this is not a concern. In any case, you will want a shallow weave for ease of maintenance.

Carpet and upholstery stains can be removed with club soda applied to the area and rubbed in a circular manner.

Hardwood floors are attractive, but expensive. The floors scratch easily, but damp-mopping, or use of a commercially available electrostatic-type Swiffer® will work well. They have to be finished, and these finishes can give off a very high level of volatile organic compounds. The volatile gases may reach one hundred times the normal indoor level depending on how much hardwood you have and how often the floor is treated and waxed.

Chapter 5
Case Histories

Case 1

A home has a leaky roof and the ceiling is wet. The wet spot moves toward a wall, where it stops. The occupant complains that there is a mold smell. The odor is heavy, and it is annoying.

While monitoring the house, you do not find mold spores in the air. The water has run down behind the wallpaper and mold growth has occurred there. Though the wallpaper has prevented the spores from entering the room, it has not prevented the smell from penetrating the paper. In this case you can locate the mold by looking for soft spots and bubbling in the wallpaper.

With a small sharp knife, cut out three sides of a rectangle about one-half inch on a side and peel it back. If mold is present you will see its black or green appearance on the wall and on the back of the paper. If it is not there, carefully replace the paper and repair it later. Continue the inspection.

Once you define the limits of the contamination, obtain some sandpaper and prepare a solution of baking soda or warm soapy water (one-half cup of baking soda per bucket of warm water). Carefully peel off the wallpaper, all the while wetting the paper with a wet sponge. This will prevent spores from entering the room. Then, wet-sandpaper the wall with a fine sandpaper, and discard the wallpaper that you removed into a plastic garbage bag. Dry the wall after removing the dark stains. Now you are now ready to repaper or repaint.

Case 2

A married couple buys an older home, and one of them complains of headaches and occasional nausea upon awakening each morning. Most of the chemicals have long since outgassed from the home. There have been no roof leaks or serious water damage and the home is in a low outdoor allergen area.

In this case, the home has a two-car garage. When a car is driven into the garage at night, the garage door is closed, thus sealing in the exhaust fumes and the greases from the heated engine. One person enters the home through a door that adjoins the kitchen, keeping the door open to bring in groceries. The fumes enter the home and are picked up by the return air register of the air-handling system, which is located just inside the kitchen door near the garage. The fumes are recirculated throughout the home, including the bedroom. Vapors from the garage also leach through the walls of the garage into the interior spaces of the home.

A good year-round compromise solution is to have a turbine fan in the roof of the garage, or an electrically operated fan, to exhaust the air of the garage. Remember that this air has to be replaced from somewhere, so you will need to create a way for the air to enter the garage from the opposite side for flow-through purposes.

Case 3

A retired couple from Michigan has been coming to their second home in balmy Florida each winter for the past twenty years. Their son has diligently maintained the home in their absence. The couple noticed that for the past five years, each of them has developed a cough within days after their arrival and lingers until after they return to their primary residence. The gas company says that the furnace is good. They have no pets, they park the car away from the house, neither has any allergies, and they live a simple life.

Under the microscope, samples of air from the home reveal high quantities of fiberglass spears bound with yellowish urea-formaldehyde. Further investigation of the home reveals an attic with old-style fiberglass cotton-like flocking that was used for insulation, and a small roof leak.

The heater and ducts are located in the attic. The duct is found to have a split at its juncture with the heater. This serves as a vacuum when air is forced through the duct; the fiberglass is not only sucked into the duct, but is sheared off to create even smaller, sharper fragments that are inhaled. A low level of mold growth is also found in the attic from the leak.

To remedy the problem, the duct has to be taped and the house has to be thoroughly damp-dusted and vacuumed. The vacuuming must be done with the windows open, and the vacuum operator should wear a mask. Once these tasks are completed, the couple ceases to have respiratory problems in this home.

Case 4

The owners of a very old mobile home do their best to maintain it. The home has leaked from time to time and is evaporative cooled during the spring and summer months. Structural textiles from within the home are no longer off-gassing formaldehyde.

During the summer, the elderly father develops a cough. His room has a window air conditioner, but this unit is found to be draining properly away from the home. The evaporative cooler is suspected of transmitting bacteria and mold into the home, but investigation clears this unit.

The father's room is found to have a high level of tiny *Aspergillus* mold spores. Once the filter on his air conditioner unit is thoroughly cleaned, his cough disappears.

Case 5

A woman lives alone and suffers from allergies to tree pollen every spring. Each April the problem becomes severe and she is reactive day and night. Her home is found to have a high level of elm pollen indoors; an elm tree is located by her bedroom window, and she states that she likes to keep that window open because she likes fresh air. It is diplomatically suggested that she try to open some windows on the opposite side of the house to see how she feels.

Case 6

After a short inspection period, a couple moves into a used home. Soon thereafter, the wife complains of allergic symptoms.

Prior to purchase, the home had been checked for the presence of mold and no contamination was found. There were no roof leaks, there was no seasonal pollen, and the climate was dry.

Her symptoms continue on a daily basis until, on a hunch, the husband requests information from the realtor regarding the lifestyle of the previous owners. The realtor informs them that the previous owners had possessed a cat.

Upon hearing this news, the wife visits her allergist, who informs her that she has a severe allergy to cat antigen.

The interior of the home is scrubbed top to bottom, including the ducts.

Within days, the wife's symptoms disappear.

Case 7

A housewife begins complaining that her periodic head-aches are getting worse. Her neighbor says that he read some-where that deadly toxic black mold could cause anything to anybody at any time. The couple checks out the home, but finds no mold.

The woman's husband thinks it might be pollen allergy. However, she has had the symptoms when pollen was not in season, and are no other symptoms of allergy present.

The woman's doctor thinks it might be a food allergy she has acquired and suggests that she not eat certain foods, in-cluding tomatoes, shellfish, nuts, and vinegar products. She does this for an extended period of time, yet finds no relief.

Fortunately, her doctor also suggests that she mark on the calendar when the headaches occur and note the correlation between them and the onset of stormy weather. She finds that there is a positive relationship between the two. (Please refer to the chapter on Weather and Your Health.)

Though there is little she can do about the weather, at least she can get back to eating the foods that she likes.

Chapter 6

Apartment Living

There are many ways that cigarette smoke, cooking odors, or indoor pesticides can travel on airways from one apartment unit to another. Whether you are the giver or the receiver, the same will apply to you.

In general, it is safe to say that odors are gases and can mix with air. As such, they can go anywhere that air can go. Any break in the wall can be an outlet or an inlet for these odors. What can the average person do at little cost with or without the permission of the management?

There are a lot of pressure changes between your unit and the one next door, or between your unit and the one above or below yours, depending on whose air conditioner or heater is on at the time. This may account for some of the smells that occur at odd hours of the day or night.

Apartments are notorious for permitting cigarette smoke or cooking odors to travel from one unit to another. There are several ways that this can happen. For example, when an exhaust fan is used in the bathroom or kitchen, negative pressure is created. This can pull in the odors. A change in pressure differential is also created when the air-conditioning or heating source is cycling between two or three different units. The use of fireplaces in condominiums and townhomes will cause an entry of outdoor air into the residence. A change in wind direction may also bring outdoor odors indoors.

One of the ways to reduce this problem, if you are the giver or receiver, is buy thin foam inserts at the hardware store that you can fit behind the wall sockets. These will work whether the outlets are used or not.

Then get some aluminum tape and seal the areas under the sinks where pipes go into the walls. Look for other areas where smoke can leave or enter your apartment. These measures will usually help.

Use tape to seal the places under the sinks or any area where pipes go into the walls. Include pipes near the water heater. If you live in a townhome or condominium, this includes the hole where the dryer hose goes through.

Aluminum tape is thinner, seals better than duct tape, and lasts longer without drying out. It is also more resistant to weather. Naturally it is going to cost more. Prices will vary but you should be able to buy foil tape at no more than 50 percent over the cost of duct tape.

Keep in mind that there is air between the walls. Electrical outlets and switches permit smells to leave or enter an apartment. Check hardware stores for electric outlet seals for receptacles and light switches. The cost is slight, and what you get is foam switch seals for your on-off switches, foam receptacle seals for your plug-ins, and safety caps to plug into unused outlets. You can unscrew the plastic switch plates yourself and simply insert these items behind them.

Take off the registers and use silicone to seal the space where the ducts are not flush against the walls. You can also use it to seal the area where lamps hang from the ceiling. Most silicone is made with acetic acid, otherwise known as vinegar, so its smell may or may not be annoying. The good news is that the odor will disappear in a short period of time.

Silicone costs between four and five dollars for a ten-ounce tube, and it comes in different colors for different purposes.

Endnotes

1. Hinds, H.C., et al. 2003 Progress Report: Relationship Between Ultrafine Particle Size Distribution and Distance from Highways. EPA Grant No. R827352C006. http://cfpub1.epa.gov/ncer_abstracts/index.cfm/fuseaction/display.abstract

2. Jones, N.C., et al. 2000. Indoor/outdoor Relationships of Particulate Matter in Domestic Homes with Roadside, Urban and Rural Locations. *Atmospheric Environ* 34(16):2603-2612.

3. Thatcher, T.L. and D.W. Layton. 1995. Deposition, Resuspension, and Penetration of Particles Within a Residence. *Atmospheric Environ* 29(13):1487-1497.

4. National Air Duct Cleaners Association. www.NADCA.com

5. Bower, J. 1989. *The Healthy House How to Buy One, How to Cure a Sick One.* Carol Communications, New York.

6. Coffel S. and K. Feiden. 1991. *A proper Airing: The Science of Ventilation. Indoor Pollution.* Ballantine Books, New York. P. 101

7. Dadd, D.L. 1986. *The Non-Toxic Home.* St. Martin's Press, NY.

8. *Chemical Residues in Animal Fibers.* Merck Veterinary Manual. Merck & Co., Inc. 2008. Whitehouse Station, New Jersey.

9. *Guide for Control of External Parasites of Sheep and Goats.* 1994 New Mexico State University. http://cahe.nmsu.edu/pubs/_b/B-112.html.

10. *Pesticide Action Network North America.* PAN Pesticides Archived October 2005. Database. http://pesticide info.org/

Bower's book is considered a classic. This comprehensive volume covers all building materials and construction practices that may have negative health effects. It lists many alternative, less toxic materials and techniques, and their suppliers.

Section 10

Selling and Buying Your Home

After inspecting and testing over five thousand homes, apartments, schools, and buildings, it is my experience that people who want to spend time in a chemically free building, whatever its nature, will find that there is no such thing.

Every residence or workplace has some type of chemical problem associated with it, whether it is part of the construction, or part of the lifestyle of the previous occupants, or as part of the ongoing nature of the business or its occupants (e.g., perfumes).

As more and more buyers express a desire to find a clean and safe residence for themselves and their children, I'd like to say that more and more realtors are becoming aware of the issues that are posed by home environments as they relate to allergies, asthma, and your sensitivity to indoor chemicals. The bad news is that many of them do not care because they need to make a sale to make a living and will make claims that are untrue, or they purport to know, but really don't. Those who have been around the block a few times and have the experience are the ones to turn to, in my experience.

The following chapters provide some basic information about what features to look for in a house, if you are buying, and how to provide those features, if you are selling.

Again, the reader is invited to review the Suggested Reading portion of the book or to browse the web, being always on the lookout for the scam artist.

Chapter 1

Preparing Your Home for Sale

There is a lot that homeowners can do to get a home as clean and fresh as possible prior to sale. Too many homes and rentals are passed by because the prior inhabitants meant well, but did the wrong things.[1,2] If you are planning to sell or lease your home, here are some tips that will help improve your chances of finding a buyer or renter.

Take a look around you. Neat and orderly is nice, but what do you smell in the various rooms? Does the bathroom reek of perfume, aftershave, chlorine bleach, and pine-scented toilet bowl cleaner? Do you have stinky cleaners and polishes under the sink? What's in the medicine cabinet? Whether you like the smells is not the issue. What you want is fresh, unscented air, because certain smells are a red flag for a lot of people, and no smell at all can mean a green light.

Normal background home smells include everything from cooking odors to personal care products, petroleum-based hydrocarbons, formaldehyde, soaps, deodorants, cleaners, paints, freshly brewed coffee, microwave popcorn, laundered and dry-cleaned clothing, and a variety of others. This background level of odors should be as low as possible when the realtor and prospective buyer walk in, or when you are absent and it is shown.

Do not use air fresheners to cover up odors. Avoid the use of scented products for cleaning purposes. Many people think that if a dab of perfume is nice, then a lot more is a lot nicer; resist this idea. Generally, the smell of perfume cannot be removed from a home. Furthermore, people with respiratory disorders will shy away from a chemically sanitized home. This group of people comprises half the population of many cities.

Frequently, the garage measures the highest hydrocarbon level in the home with readings of more than seven parts per million (ppm) when the background level of the home is usually 0.2-0.3 ppm. If it is oil-stained, the garage floor can be scrubbed down with a solution of 5 percent trisodium phosphate (TSP) (about two ounces per quart of water). TSP is odor free and will remove the grease and attendant odors. Extremely inexpensive, it is available in hardware stores and can be used for the cleaning of laundry room and under sink shelves as well. (Please refer to the section on Safe Household Cleaning.)

The laundry room should be clean of old soap residue on the washer and dryer and on the floor. Check behind the units. These areas are usually laden with dust, soap residue, antistatic sheets, and lost personal items. Wash the shelves with your TSP solution (use gloves) or baking soda to remove the smells of chlorine bleach, detergent, pine scent, fabric softeners, antistatic products, paint thinner, shoe polish, furniture polish, and pesticides. This area is a hot spot where outgassing occurs into the rest of the home and is sure to annoy some potential buyer.

If you want to wash the walls and countertops, you can use a half cup of baking soda in a bucket of warm water. You will be surprised how inexpensive and effective it can be.

There is nothing wrong with cleaning the home and then going away to leave it in the hands of a realtor to lease or sell. There is, however, a problem with having the carpets cleaned and shampooed and then locking up the house. Allow enough time for the carpets to dry. Otherwise residual moisture from the carpets will aerosolize any smells that they have absorbed.

These homes frequently smell bad when they are opened (sometimes weeks and months later), and it is very difficult to remove the odor at that point because it has become part of the walls and ceiling.

From the realtors' standpoint, idle homes need to be completely opened and aired out on occasion anyway, and not just when there is a showing. At that point it may be too late. I have been with an all cash paying client who walked away from a sale for just this reason.

The air-conditioning or heating filter should be changed prior to showing in case some mechanically minded person wants to look at it. Besides, the presence of clean filters suggests that the home is cared for. It's like having clean oil in a car that is for sale.

For desert dwellers, the evaporative cooler should be cleaned and serviced prior to sale so that it is quiet and works efficiently.

If possible, keep your pets out of the home when potential buyers are present. People who are concerned about allergies do not like to see pet food or pet toys or have animals running around and jumping on them. They are looking for a home that is going to be good to them.

The use of too much wood polish can raise the concentration of volatile organic compounds to an irritating level of as much as fifteen ppm. This can kill a sale.

Obviously, the yard and the alley need to be kept trim to reduce the incidence of allergenic pollen from weeds and grass. If you have a lawn, it is a no-win situation for an allergic or asthmatic person, as all grasses are allergenic to some degree. This means their cuttings, as well.

Chapter 2
Buying a Home: Outdoor Factors

Regardless of where you choose to live, you will have to deal with the outdoor environment. The issue could be diesel exhaust carbon, ozone, or pollen or mold. But exposure to allergens and irritants can still be minimized with a little homework.

First, it will be very helpful for you to know the prevailing wind direction during the spring and fall months. Paying attention to your local weather service, radio, or television newscaster can help, as can simple awareness and common sense. Unfortunately, this factor may be different in different locales within the city due to the presence of mountains or manmade structures. The latter can result in drafting and wind channeling.

Next, it is helpful to know which you are sensitive to: pollen, mold, or dust. This knowledge will help determine what side of the city you may want to live on. For example, suppose you are sensitive to tree pollen of all types, and the prevailing springtime breezes are from the south. In that case, you may want to find a residence on the south side (upwind from the trees of your city), if that is possible. If you are sensitive predominantly to fall weed and grass pollen and the fall breezes come from the north, then you may want to reside on the north end of the city, unless there are weedy areas immediately to the north of the home. The concentration of airborne pollen is highest nearest the source, although admittedly, it doesn't take much of the allergen to trigger a response in most pollen-sensitive patients.

Lower parts of the city and cooler temperatures in the morning hours bring particles in the atmosphere downward to settle out because of the denser air. Thus, you may need to avoid areas that are significantly lower in elevation, or just don't open the windows at night for fresh air.

The residence itself should have a minimum of vegetation immediately around it to reduce the amount of local mold and pollen. Each home has a microbial shell around it that is influenced primarily by the local vegetation, secondarily by neighboring vegetation, and finally by distant vegetation. Lawns are scarce in some communities. If that is the case for yours, pay attention to the type of landscaping that your neighbors have. If there is a lawn associated with the residence, expect your exposure to a wide variety of allergenic grass particles and mold to be elevated. Incidentally, that includes a well-kept lawn. Who is going to cut the grass?

Living in the country is a virtual guarantee that you will be exposed to a high concentration of pollen and mold from the local vegetation. Not only that, but expect it to become tracked into the home on shoes and boots. This includes the kitchen and dining room, sitting room, and master bedroom.

Learn your trees. Watch for trees that are too close to windows of the residence. Or, if trees are next to a main walkway, they will shed pollen that, once again, can be tracked indoors.

You may also wish to find out if any major road construction will be taking place in your prospective new area or residence, as this means tar fumes, diesel smoke, and outdoor dust may be present for a long time. Your city planning and zoning department can help you here. Do not rely on your realtor for this information. This is not his or her area of expertise.

In inner-city neighborhoods, look over the back fence of the residence. Is the alley clean, or is it full of grass and weeds that nobody except you will ever cut?

Find out the average amount of rainfall for the city you wish to move to. The number of aeroallergens is generally related to rainfall. More rainfall means more plants, more pollen, and more molds.

If you are looking at apartment units, watch for piles of swirling dust on certain doorsteps. This is a clue that channel drafting is occurring, and that the residence is at the end of a natural or manmade channel (such as between buildings). Wind will travel down these channels and carry debris. This will cause a much higher rate of buildup of allergenic particles within the building and increase your exposure level.

There is evidence that any kind of windbreak will significantly reduce the exposure of your residence to allergenic substances being carried on the wind. This means that a stand of insect-pollinated trees, a fence, or another building can help redirect the flow of particles away from you. The use of a stand of oleanders is questioned because of the poisonous nature of the plant and its attendant litter.

No residence or area is going to be perfect. Be prepared to make tradeoffs.

Chapter 3

Buying a Home: Indoor Factors

Weather stripping has its good and bad points. On the plus side, it keeps out dust and aeroallergens and increases energy efficiency of the home. This saves money. On the minus side, it does not permit the home to breathe. A home needs to be ventilated with fresh air to reduce the buildup of a variety of indoor pollutants, as discussed in other sections.

The level of indoor humidity will vary greatly from day to day and season to season, and it will have to be controlled with a dehumidifier or other methods to keep down mold growth and the proliferation of dust mites., one of the top allergens that we have to face. The amount of weatherproofing you do will depend on your level of sensitivity to outdoor or indoor pollutants. You can check with your local home builders' association for recommendations in this regard.

Look for fan ventilation in the bathrooms and kitchen. The presence of a fan not only permits the reduction of moisture buildup in the bathroom, but is instrumental in the removal of volatile organic compounds that are generated through the use of personal care products. This is also true for the stove top fan.

Find out if there have been any water leaks indoors. There are a half-a-hundred ways that virtually any home anywhere in the country can incur water damage so it is important to know this fact. Many states now have disclosure laws in this regard.

If the carpets and baseboards have not been thoroughly

dried within two to three days after a water loss, there may be a real mold problem. Mold species such as *Aspergillus, Penicillium, Stachybotrys, Phoma, Cladosporium,* and several others are likely culprits. All of these are potentially allergenic species to your family, houseguests, and pets.

When you first inspect your potential new home or apartment, look for stains on the ceiling, walls, floor, and carpet, and try to find out what caused them. Has the roof leaked? Is the bathroom unvented? Usually, the presence of ceiling stains does not mean that spores are in the airspace, although they may be present above the ceiling. Their presence above the ceiling or within the walls does not usually pose a problem in regards to the airspace inside the dwelling.

Many attics serve as storage areas or living areas. They may provide a space for ductwork and may have fiberglass flocking as insulation. If so, there is an even chance that materials contaminated from a roof leak or fiberglass particles are gaining entrance into the home proper. (Please refer to the chapter on Fiberglass.) True attics have their own microbial ecosystem and microclimate and should be insulated from the ceiling of the home below them. Check to see if an attic exhaust fan is present.

Basements are a major issue because of their history of musty odors, mold growth, high humidity, and the possible presence of water from window leakage or a break in the hot water heater. Radon gas may be a possible resident of the basement.

Ideally the basement should be ventilated to remove radon and a floor drain for the drainage of moisture from the dehumidifier. In today's electronic world, remote humidity-sensing devices are available to alert family members of the condition of the attic or basement through inspection of the gauges located within the home proper.

Check out the laundry room. If you are annoyed by fragrances and chemical smells, then you are going to have to scrub out this area when you move in.

Does the refrigerator come with the home? Then it may have to be inspected and decontaminated.

Check the condition of the fireplace and the operation of the damper.

What kind of filter is being used in the central air-handling system? If they are the standard fiberglass variety, you will need to upgrade to a pleated filter.

Note the relative location of the garage, carport, or parking area with respect to the home. If there is an attached garage, is a return air duct located by the entry? This could be a source of auto exhaust into the entire home. You may need to weather strip this door thoroughly.

Homes that have shade on all sides have potential for mold buildup. Try to find a home that has a reasonable amount of exposure to natural light.

(If you do buy the home, plan to minimize the tracking of particles indoors by placing a quality shoe mat outside each entry to the home. These outdoor mats can go a long way toward lessening this potential problem, if taking off your shoes upon entry is not compatible with your lifestyle.)

Finally, in addition to walking around to just get the feel of the place, you may want to prepare a checklist before you inspect your potential new residence.

Suggested Reading

1. Hunter, L.M.1990. *The Healthy Home: An Attic-to-Basement Guide to Toxin-Free Living*. Pocket Books, NY.

2. Bower, J. 1989. *The Healthy House: How to Buy One, How to Cure a Sick One*. Carol Communications, New York

3. Dadd, D.L. 1986. *The Nontoxic Home: Protecting Yourself and Your Family from Everyday Toxics and Health Hazards*. Tarcher, Inc. Los Angeles.

4. NIOSH Pocket Guide to Chemical Hazards, U.S. Department of Human and Health Services, Centers for Disease Control and Prevention, 1997. Publ. No. 97-140

Section 11

Schools

According to EPA-sponsored Tools for Schools seminars held around the country,[1] one-third of the nation's schools have indoor air quality (IAQ) problems, and asthma is on the increase. (Please see the section on Asthma.) Poor IAQ means that the rate and the amount of learning decreases. There are a variety of reasons for this. As investigations continue, more useful information has become available. Some of it may surprise you.[2]

According to the National Center for Education Statistics:[3]

There were 95,726 public schools in the U.S. during the 2003-2004 school year.

There were over 34 million K-8 public school students and another ten percent (approximately) K-8 private school students.

In the grades 9-12, there were over 15 million public school students and approximately ten percent of this number in the same grades at the private school level.

About 1.2 million students were enrolled in 4,132 charter schools in 2006-2007.

Attendance in schools by males and females is about equal

up through age 17, after which the percentage of females decreases slightly.[4]

Disease Transmission in Schools:

(Please see the chapter on The Spread of Viruses and Bacteria.)

A school administrators' article pointedly notes that handwashing cuts germs and abseentism.[5]

Careful handwashing at school four times daily can result in 24 percent fewer colds and 50 percent fewer illnesses at daycare, as well as reduced stomach problems.[6] This is due to removal of cold and flu viruses and intestinal bacteria, as long as quality handwashing is instituted. Not surprisingly, there is a right way and a wrong way to wash hands. The websites provide this information, which is beyond the scope of this book.

Repeatedly, evidence has demonstrated that alcohol-based hand washes are more effective than soap and water for the removal of terms, when handwashing is done properly. Indeed, according to the United States Department of Health and Human Services Centers for Disease Control and Prevention, *proper* handwashing and use of alcohol-based hand rubs has been shown to reduce overall infection rates.[6,7,8]

Thus, without launching into statistics regarding the reduction in virus and bacterial transmission of disease causing agents, it is clear that ample data demonstrate significant reduction in school absenteeism from the standpoint of students, teachers, and faculty with this simple practice. Why don't we do it more?

Would not the average school benefit greatly from a financial and educational sense if an IAQ walk-around was conducted, proper handwashing was practiced upon return from recess, and an honest attempt was made to reduce the transmission of disease through the use of fomites?

The cost of alcohol-base handwashes is minimal when compared with the cost of dollars lost to the average school due to sick days.

A serious discussion regarding the reduction of asthma triggers in schools is offered.[9]

Chapter 1

Why Schools Have
Air Quality Problems

I recommend walk-through inspections to detail and prioritize problems in terms of effect and cost to remediate.

This walk-through will be beneficial for a number of reasons:

1. Why aren't walk-throughs conducted? They don't cost anything, and they can save money for the school and the district in many ways, In addition, many, if not most states, school districts get grant monies for attendance.

2. Children are more susceptible than adults to respiratory irritants and allergens.

3. Schools are four times more crowded than office buildings.

4. Renovating activities put children and staff at risk because the practices utilized are almost always mishandled by contractors.

5. Budgets are tight, so low-bid contractors are hired for all phases of work.

6. School boards and administrators typically have a re-

active rather than proactive policy in dealing with air-quality issues.

7. Room configurations change along with activity levels, and this affects the air quality and the ability of the air-handling system to provide enough fresh air to the areas that have the most children.

8. Energy control is centralized and often out of the teachers' hands.

9. Sometimes there are different ventilation systems in the same school, so different air-quality issues have to be addressed.

10. There are unique topics that need to be dealt with separately; for example, gym, art class, shops, exhaust from motor vehicles, lawn care, trees on campus, and after-hours room maintenance.

11. Poor pest management.

12. Slow response to complaints; problems get worse, people polarize and become sensitized and hostile, and the press gets involved.

13. The location of the fresh air supply can be near a sewer outlet, diesel engine supply trucks, school buses, or dumpsters.

Chapter 2

Back to School

Direct observation (and awareness) of potential problem areas followed by action can have a positive impact on students' ability to learn.

There are many respiratory-related issues of concern to the school district, teachers, staff, parents, and ultimately the students. These include nontoxic art supplies, the lawn cutting schedule, pesticide use and abuse, idling school buses, delivery vehicles, and parental cars that park near air intakes. Other issues include the presence of asbestos (usually a perceived problem rather than a real one), carpeting versus tile floors, pollen-producing weeds, trees and grass on and around the school grounds, contaminated air-handling systems, and piles of chalk dust that act as an irritant.

There's more: vapors from the laminating press, mimeograph fluid (still used by many poorer school districts) and toxic xylene-based markers, odors of sewer gas from dry plumbing traps, indoor mold growth and mite contamination, cat antigen (figure it to be always present), outgassing of structural materials from newly remodeled rooms, and finally, as always, the unknown.

Teachers comprise the largest group of professionals that complain of chemical sensitivity. This has been attributed to the fact that they stay in one location all day and are exposed to herbicides and pesticides that are used in and around the schools.

For concerned parents, it is helpful to know that some progress has been made in recent years to clean up the schools. For example, virtually all schools now carry EPA-approved cleaning chemicals. Schools are also aware of the problems that revolve around new carpeting and the necessity of maintaining fresh air ventilation. Nontoxic art supplies are coming to the fore to replace xylene-containing solvents that had been in use by millions of people for decades.

Learning increases when the teachers and students are not suffering from poor air quality. Private schools and school districts around the country are aware of these potential health hazards. Unfortunately, just because there is awareness does not always mean there is change.

For parents whose children have respiratory problems, it's necessary to stay in touch with the school nurse and with their doctor. The asthmatic child can still exercise if the supervising teacher and nurse are aware of the problem and precautionary measures are taken. Many Olympic athletes have allergies and asthma and still train for hours a day, competing at a world-class level.

If we expect our children's school to be safe, then the home environment also must be maintained in a clean manner. Responsibility has to be shared.

Chapter 3

Special Classes Have Special Needs

Climate conditions do not always lend themselves to fresh air ventilation. Two other solutions regarding the dilution of indoor air include the use of an exhaust fan and a switch to less toxic materials.

Teachers' prep room

Many prep rooms are poorly ventilated. They lack newer and less toxic equipment.

Photocopy machines are frequently small and poorly ventilated. They may release a high concentration of ozone gas, a strong lung irritant. Long-term exposure to ozone at a high concentration may cause chronic bronchitis. (Please refer to the chapter on Ozone.)

A few schools still use ditto or mimeograph machines. These present a respiratory hazard due to the fluid that contains high concentrations of methanol (methyl alcohol). Exposure to methanol can cause headaches, dizziness, nausea, and blurred vision unless adequate ventilation is in place.[10]

Good ventilation and use of duplicating fluid that contains less than 5 percent methanol will resolve this problem. Also, allow dittos to dry before handling and distribution, as methanol can be absorbed through the skin.

Respiratory irritation can occur from carbonless copy paper and typing correction fluid that is not water- based.

Older-style laminating presses are immediately toxic when they release gases from the heated laminated plastic.

Art room

In the art room, a spray booth should be used when spraying ceramic glazes or airbrushing with paints. Aerosol spray fixatives should only be used outdoors or in an explosion-proof spray booth. Pastel chalks will powder and can be inhaled.

Dilution ventilation, such as a window or roof exhaust fan, is recommended when using certain materials. These materials include rubber cement or permanent markers that release a small amount of solvents. Water-based markers are now available at almost all supply stores.

Vocational classes

In vocational classes, problems may arise where cars are sanded and spray painted; older brakes are repaired with exposure to asbestos; cars are idling indoors exposing persons to carbon monoxide; photographic chemicals are not exhausted (this also happens in hospitals where X-ray development machines are located in hallways or near waiting rooms); and printing inks contain solvents and pigments, which can be inhaled or enter through the skin.

Students who work in woodworking classes are exposed to formaldehyde outgassing from adhesives. These are found in plywood and particle board, fine sand, wood and varnish particles during the sanding process, and the vapors from varnishes used to complete a project.

Chapter 4

Vo-Tech Schools—Almost All Have Their Problems

There is an increasing national interest in the indoor air quality at schools. This is of no surprise when we consider the increase in the incidence of respiratory problems, dermatitis, and chemical sensitivity over the past few years. Tens of thousands of pages have been written on this subject.

What I say also applies to homes and to the hobbyist who spends his or her time in that enclosed and confined location called the 'special room' or the garage.

Chief among the problem schools are the vocational-technical, also known as Vo-Tech schools. These include strictly Vo-Tech schools, those associated with public schools, and special classes offered by city parks and recreation departments. The real problem is the lack of awareness of what is happening. We can also call it a lack of education.

In many Vo-Tech schools, old-school attitudes still prevail:

» The chemicals that we smell won't hurt you; after all, I've smelled them for years and I'm okay.

» This is all that is available.

» These are the materials the student will work with in the professional world so he or she can get used to them.

» Sawdust is just wood, and the pieces are too big to breathe. (99.99 percent of the dust is actually one micron or less in size and will get to the deeper lungs immediately).[11]

» Asthma is caused by allergies and not by paint solvents.

» Even if we wanted to fix the problem, we don't have the money.

Improvements can be made in any Vo-Tech school when people want to make improvements.

Though money is always an issue, lack of money should not be a fallback excuse. There are low-budget solutions to many of the problems.

Let us enumerate just some of the issues that need to be addressed: spray paint fumes, powerful cleaning solvents, acid-washes, welding and soldering, auto exhaust, auto body putties and body fillers, concentrated levels of airborne sawdust, cosmetology materials, paint solvents, photography development chemicals, engine repair and degreasers, improper storage of chemicals, metal grinding and metal fabrication, improper room air pressure balance, lack of adequate ventilation in buildings, and overcrowded buildings.

One of the biggest problems in the Vo-Tech school arena and in the business world as well, is the autobody shop. These concerns are environmentally based and worker related. Workers in autobody shops are potentially exposed to a variety of chemical and physical hazards. These include volatile organic compounds (VOCs) from paints, fillers and solvents, silica from sandblasting operations; chromium from spray painting, dusts from sanding; and metal fumes from welding and cutting.[12] According to NIOSH, exposure to isocyanates could lead to irritation, asthma, hypersensitivity pneumonitis, and cancer. Inhalation of vapor or aerosols occurs through use of spray paints, but physical contact with solvents is also hazardous.[13]

A newer problem is the use of the laser for cutting materials. I have monitored air in which a laser is used to cut plastic. Microscopic globules of plastic fill the air.

Though they may appear sterile, computer labs also fit into the problem category. In my experience, the level of VOCs in these arenas is always elevated. One reason is that the electronic equipment emits VOCs. Another is that the rooms are enclosed, with poor ventilation. When many people are in such rooms, their personal care products add to the concentration of VOCs in the air.

Where gases are concerned, such as chemical smells and exhaust, fresh air dilution and point source control will help. For instance, improperly closed containers of chemicals and solvents contribute to the irritant vapors in the air. Ensuring that containers are closed and their tops cleaned is a form of point-source control. Wipe and spill rags need to be kept out of the main airstream. Store them in compliance with fire safety codes.

If a window exhaust fan is installed, this can make a big difference. Ducting can be rigged with an exhaust fan near a work area to carry out contaminated air. This works best when there is a supply of fresh air to replace the air that is exhausted from the building.

One problem with the venting of exhaust air is its ultimate destination. Is it going to another room or another building? It might be better to vent it through the roof. Even a bathroom fan that is left on will help remove polluted air.

Dust masks are readily available from a number of companies. They are made for industry, trade school, and home usage. They are constructed to remove particles or gases or both. Their cost should be included as part of enrollment fees.

Chapter 5

What You Can Do to Improve the IAQ of Your School at Little or No Cost

School administrations tend to be weighed down by problems other than IAQ, so make long-term plans and not immediate radical changes.

To assess the magnitude of a school's problems, take a walk-through with the checklist below in hand. There will be fewer sick days if the air of the school is clean. Learning will improve and because many schools receive state funds for attendance, funding will also increase.

Not all of these suggestions are practical for each school. However, teachers have strong propensity for learning new things, including information that will improve the quality of their own lives.

- Be very careful of renovation activities. Recommend the use of paints that have a low VOC level and suggest ways to protect students and staff from work dust.

- Evaluate present pest-management policies and adopt integrated pest management techniques.

- Remove old carpeting, where practical, to ensure ease of floor cleaning and replace with area rugs, when appropriate.

- Examine special use areas such as shops and art studios; evaluate teachers' prep rooms to determine if there is enough fresh air to dilute the effects of equipment such as ditto (mimeograph) machines, laminating presses, and copiers; this includes offices with numerous pieces of electronic equipment.

- If necessary, reschedule lawn cutting and indoor and outdoor pesticide usage for afterschool hours,

- Improve vacuuming techniques and use upgraded bags.

- Utilize damp dusting, including chalk trays; be aware of dust that will settle on cabinets above eye level.

- Place large (five-square-foot) shoe-scrub mats outside outer doors to reduce indoor particle load.

- If fresh air intakes are located downwind from buses, delivery trucks, or garbage dumpsters, make the necessary adjustments to the problem sources.

- Replace air handling filters on or before schedule and see if upgraded filters can be adapted to your air-handling system.

- Open windows for fresh air when possible. This may not be possible during pollen and mold season or during winter months.

- Obtain nontoxic art supplies such as water-base markers and glues.

- Ensure that p-traps that enter sewer lines are full of water.

- Cut back pollen-producing trees that are close to doors and windows.

- Ask maintenance staff to check classroom size versus airflow to ensure there is enough fresh air for room configuration and activities (twenty cubic feet per minute per occupant is recommended).

- Clean the grills on the supply and return air registers in the classrooms if they are discolored; this discoloration is frequently due to mold growth on the paint.

- Minimize the use of scented personal care products and bathroom fragrances.

- Discuss these issues as a regular part of staff meetings to improve attendance and include a discussion about proper handwashing to reduce rate of sick days of teachers and students. (Please refer to the introduction to this section and to the chapter on The Spread of Viruses and Bacteria.)

- Utilize EPA-approved cleaning supplies, including floor waxes, and ensure that dirty mops are not left in hallways.

- Be very careful about what is used to clean drinking fountains.

- Collect anonymous suggestions from teachers and students regarding IAQ complaints.

- Check that jars, cans and bottles of varnishes, cleaners,

stains, polishes, and other toxic materials are tightly sealed, labeled, and stored properly.

- Report moisture damage and mold contamination immediately; note any change in the health status of children and staff in the affected room or area. Periodically check for damp areas on ceiling tiles as a sign of roof leaks, and check behind bookcases or wall charts and photographs where humidity is the highest.

- Indoor pollutants may be linked to a sudden increase in behavioral or learning problems. This is especially true when VOCs are a source of the problem.

- Weather-strip doors and windows.

- If the gym floor needs to be stripped, varnished, and waxed, this exercise should be conducted at the start of a one-to-two week vacation period or longer; allow for an abundance of fresh air and ensure that there is a maximum amount of exhaust air,

- Teach your students to practice good habits related to IAQ for their own growth and development.

Chapter 6

Summary: Air Quality Status of our Nation's Schools

Ten million school days are lost each year due to allergy and asthma, and one-third of the nation's schools have IAQ problems. Wouldn't learning improve if we could cut back on these lost days? What if we could solve many of the problems at no cost?

Microbial problems occur when there is water damage. And this is made worse by poor repair and lack of adequate planning during remodeling as pertains to air quality.

When the public passes a bond issue to add to or improve one or more schools, it's typical for a contractor to be hired who has been working on schools for many years, but who has no concept of IAQ.

Typically, ceiling tiles will be removed that have been in place for decades. The ceiling tiles will contain water-associated gram-negative bacteria that cause flulike symptoms through the presence of their endotoxins, along with all manner of mold genera that have grown as a result of roof leakage over the years. These fungi will be allergenic. Expect to find a high concentration of dust, dust mites, and dust mites' allergenic feces, along with allergenic plant parts and a very high concentration of diesel exhaust carbon.

New carpeting will be installed, and painting and varnishing will occur. This work frequently takes place while school is in session. Students and staff will become ill, but it will be several months to a year or more before an IAQ expert is called in to investigate reported problems.

The sequence of events continues: Somebody will complain about an illness at the school. The school or district will ignore the complaint. Other people become ill, parents become concerned, the press and lawyers get called in, a superficial approach is taken by the school or district, parents become outraged, and what was once a small problem now becomes a major issue.

What this tells us is that an IAQ complaint should be investigated quickly to minimize liability issues, and an IAQ expert should be part of the remodeling team.

Chapter 7
Volatile Organic Compounds Cause Behavioral and Learning Problems

Most people are familiar with the classic symptoms of allergy such as sneezing, coughing, and itching and watering eyes. We are also familiar with reactions to chemicals that include headaches and eye irritation. However, researchers are now also looking at the effects of aeroallergens and chemical pollutants on behavior.

Behavioral changes can occur in students within a matter of minutes after exposure to chemical irritants. (This may also occur in adults—Please refer to the chapter on Perfumes and Fragrances.) In children, these changes include acting out, changes in handwriting, and changes in drawing patterns, the use of foul language, throwing tantrums, exhibiting unprovoked aggression, and drowsiness. They can occur after a child eats a meal that contains an allergenic food. They can also occur when a child smells a marker with xylene, a school-cleaning agent that contains phenol, or volatile byproducts of mold growth. Many of them have hydrocarbons and benzene rings. (Please refer to the chapter on Mold Smell.)

Let's look at handwriting as an example. According to Doris J. Rapp, MD, [14] a child tends to write from right to left or increase the size of letters after exposure. Letters become poorly written. Hyperactive children write with large letters. Withdrawn children begin writing smaller letters, or they refuse to write at all. Aggressive children write with abandon, hostility, anger, and violence.

Pictures children draw become hostile, dark, and violent in nature, or they may be abstract. Children who were able to color between the lines before exposure might lose this ability.

If the problem begins during or after a rainy day, then allergic sensitivity to mold or pollen may be the problem (thunderstorm asthma). If it occurs after the child returns from the lavatory (or the drinking fountain), it may be a reaction to cleaning agents used by the janitorial staff. If it happens after lunch, then there may be a food or drink sensitivity. It could be any food or drink, but dyes are frequently to blame. If it happens after a ride on the school bus, then diesel or auto exhaust may be the problem.

Teachers and staff should be alerted to watch for drawing and writing skills that suddenly decline, or behavior that takes a fast downturn. They will frequently discover the cause of the problem. Elimination of the problem will allow for improved learning.

Water-based markers are readily available, and schools should endeavor to constantly improve their use of nontoxic cleaning supplies.

We are learning a lot about our school environment and ways to change it for the better at little or no cost.

Obviously, what is presented above may apply to adults, depending on their level of sensitivity.

Endnotes

1. EPA. 2002. *Indoor Air Quality Tools for Schools Program: Benefits of Improving Air Quality in the School Environment.* Office of Air & Radiation Indoor Environments Division. Doc 402-K-02-005 Oct.

2. EPA. 1996. *Indoor Air Quality Basics for Schools.* Indoor Environments Division EPA document 402-F-96-004 Oct.

3. U.S. Department of Education National Center for Education Statistics. www.NCES.ed.gov

4. U.S. Department of Commerce Bureau of the Census from Digest of Education Statistics 2004. http://www.infoplease.com/us/census/enrolled-in-school-2004.html

5. Minnesota Department of Health. *Handwashing Gets Results.* www.health.state.mm.us/handhygiene/schools/results

6. St. Mary Medical Center. *Handwashing Facts and Tips.* www.st-maryhealthcare.org/body.cfm?id=555953.

7. Education World. *Germs Spread into School Cirriculum: Handwashing Saves the Day.* http://www.educationworld.com/a_curr/curr016 as reported by the Centers for the CDC

8. CDC Handwashing. http://www.cdc.gov/handhygiene/

9. *Reducing Asthma Triggers in Schools: Recommendations for Effective Policies, Regulations, and Legislation.* Asthma Regional Council of New England. www.asthmaregional council.org/about/documents/Reducing AsthmaTriggersinSchools.pdf

10. NIOSH Pocket Guide to Chemical Hazards, U.S. Department of Human and Health Services, Centers for Disease Control and Prevention, 1997. Publ. No. 97-140

11. LSU AgCenter. 2006. *Sawmill Sawdust Particle Size vs. Potential Effects on Health.* http://text.lsuagcenter.com/en/environment/forestry/forest_products/Is+Sawmill+Sawdust+Dangerous.htm

12. United States Department of Labor, Occupational Safety and Health. *Autobody Repair and Finishing* www.osha.gov/SLTC/autobody/iindex.html.

13. *NIOSH Warns of Asthma, Death from Diisocyanate Exposure in the Auto Industry.* www.search-autoparts.com/searchautoparts/articleDetail.jsp?id=159210

14. Rapp, D. 1996. Handwriting and Drawing Changes. *In: Is This Your Child's World?* Bantam Books, New York 78-114

Section 12

Mold

Mold belongs to the family of fungi. Simply put, they require only oxygen, water, and nutrition to survive. These fungi include an extremely diverse group of life forms.

Molds appear virtually everywhere, indoors and outdoors. They have been found on the surface of rocks in the world's greatest deserts, from the Gobi to the Mojave to the Kalahari.

Mold is different from radon, asbestos, and lead. It is biological in origin and can reproduce at a moment's notice. Microscopically, it can be seen to produce its string-like strands within seconds, once moisture is added to spores. Some of the life forms can produce airborne spores at the touch of a raindrop.

The integration of mold in our lives cannot be underestimated, from the production of antibiotics to the destruction of crops worldwide, to the manufacture of alcohol and bread, to the symptoms of allergy and asthma.

In this section, I present a comprehensive and informative guide to mold as it affects our daily outdoor and indoor lives. Nothing too exotic, but the exotic is there if one wishes to further explore this universe.

Chapter 1

Effects of Mold on Health

Mold can adversely affect us in a number of ways: Inhaling their spores can cause allergic symptoms, asthmatic reactions and lung infections. Their odors may act as an asthma trigger. Toxic poisoning can occur if one eats mushrooms, ergot-containing grains, or mycotoxin-contaminated foodstuffs such as rice, peanuts, and soy products. Vaginal and oral infections may occur from the yeast *Candida albicans*, disseminated infections can occur due to fungi associated with birds and soil (histoplasmosis, blastomycosis, and coccidioidomycosis). Invasion of the bones and muscles and organ systems can occur in more tropical climates by a variety of exotic pathogenic fungi.

The good news is that fungal usage also yields many beneficial products, including vinegar, yeasts that produce alcoholic beverages, and the yeasts used in the baking industry that cause bread to rise. Many fungi also produce antibiotics, including penicillin and cyclosporin and have saved millions of lives.

The general classification of fungi includes the common mold and mildew. Mildew is a vernacular term that refers to mold growth on clothing and usually includes many of the same genera that contaminate structural materials. The grouping of fungi also includes mushrooms, and a spectrum of exotic forms that infect humans around the world.

Fungal infections and deep mycotic diseases pose a greater risk for the very young, the elderly, and those who have an immunologic deficiency. These include people who have a depressed immune system for a number of reasons—for instance, the presence of HIV or other viruses, a low white blood cell count, chemotherapy, and heavy doses of steroids.

Unlike radon and asbestos, which take decades to show an effect on people, or lead, which can take a few years to affect the learning process, mold can produce immediate effects.

The most common complaints relating to exposure to everyday mold spores includes symptoms of allergy and asthma, where sneezing, itching and watering eyes, nasal congestion, sinus drainage, coughing, and other symptoms of allergy are commonplace. Headaches, loss of concentration, rashes, and other nervous symptom reactions are extremely rare after exposure to mold spores.

The greater one's exposure to mold, the greater the risk of infection. And like pollen, the risk of infection increases as the number of infection agents and the strength of the infection agent increases.

Science cannot yet measure the effect of toxins at a low concentration on people exposed to mold. This is because the toxins have only recently been associated with mold spores. Additionally, nobody knows how many spores or how much toxin can cause a person to react, particularly when the person's state of health varies from day to day. There is also insufficient data available to link inhalation of mold spores with health effects related to mold.

The scientific literature reports deaths in people who have been exposed to spores from various species of *Aspergillus* during renovation of hospitals. The spores come from areas that were previously contaminated due to water damage. If the areas are torn down (e.g., dropped ceilings) and isolation of the area does *not* occur, spores will enter the wings where cancer patients and other immunocompromised persons are housed.

Similarly, schools find themselves in trouble when protection is not afforded to the student body or the staff during renovation activities. In these cases, common symptoms of allergy can occur.

Diseases

Depending on how one defines the term disease, there are perhaps fifty or more fungal diseases that occur around the world.

Stachybotrys has received a lot of publicity because of its implication in human lung disease. This fungus produces toxins known as mycotoxins (from *mycos*, which is Greek for fungus). This is not surprising in that virtually all of the common fungi produce mycotoxins under the right conditions. The fact that these toxins actually cause harm to humans when the spores are inhaled is debatable and has yet to be proved to the satisfaction of major medical organizations.

Candida albicans causes a disease known as candidiasis, a common yeast infection familiar to tens of millions of women. This infection, among others has brought about the use of antibiotics that may be prescribed to cure another intestinal infection.

Another common mold causes ringworm. Three related fungi also cause this problem; the disease is prevalent in more humid areas of the United States, and is particularly common in other parts of the world.

The ringworm fungi have a predilection for keratin, found in human skin cells, nails, and hair, and in animal hooves.

Almost unique among fungal diseases, ringworm can spread from person-to-person by contact and from one area of the body to another by scratching. In short, it is a communicable fungal disease.

Circular patches of ringworm on the hair and skin, frequently accompanied by itching, are the signatures of this disease, but mold growth can occur between the toes and in the groin area, as testified by soldiers who fought in a variety of wars in tropical countries. The disease is commonly contracted by men and women who frequent locker rooms in the gymnasiums, or by horticulturalists who dig with bare hands in soils where animal hair is prominent. It may also be contracted by persons who wear boots or shoes for a number of days where the footwear lacks adequate ventilation.

Hypersensitivity pneumonitis is inflammation of the lungs due to breathing in a foreign substance, usually certain types of dust, fungi, or molds. The most common molds associated with the disease belong to the *Aspergillus* or *Penicillium* genera although numerous fungi including yeasts can be involved. It is also known as Farmer's lung, humidifier lung or greenhouse pneumonitis.

Exposure to moldy hay, peat moss, moldy cork dust, wood dust, mist from hot tubs, infested flour, and numerous other sources may bring about the disease.

"Hypersensitivity Pneumonitis" by Cecile Rose in (Murray) Hypersensitivity Pneumonitis and Organic Dust Toxic Syndromes" by Yvon Cormer and Mark Schuyler in (Asthma in the Workplace)

Diphasic Fungi

There are several fungi within the United States and the world that are classed as diphasic, that is, their spores have one appearance in the ground or in culture, but convert to another type once inhaled. The names of these are rather cumbersome. Three of the most cumbersome names include the following: Ohio or Mississippi River Valley Fever or histoplasmosis (histo); the Chicago disease or blastomycosis (blasto); and San Joaquin Valley Fever caused by *Coccidioides immitis* (cocci).

These diseases affect infect large numbers of persons annually and are usually benign in their symptomotology. However, they have the ability to spread throughout the body.

Histoplasmosis is known as Mississippi River or Ohio River Valley Fever. The full name of the fungus is *Histoplasma capsulatum*. The fungus is found in over sixty countries in soil that is enriched by the droppings of starlings (that frequent trees), chickens, and other birds, as well as bats. Wind blown spores result in their inhalation and a possible infective state.

The disease is usually asymptomatic when in the lungs. However, if the disease spreads throughout the body, it may occur in all age groups. The spores will change into a yeast-like form in the body and may infect various cells in the lungs, spleen, liver, adrenals, kidneys, skin, central nervous system and other organs. The dog and other animals may also become infected.

Blastomycosis, also known as Chicago's disease, also begins in the respiratory tract. Its causative agent is *Blastomyces dermatitidis*. Once the fungal spores of this agent convert to another form, they may spread to the bones and skin.

The disease is found with the largest numbers in the Mississippi Valley and the southeastern United States, as well as in Africa. It is occasionally found in Canada and Central America. Similar to histoplasmosis, the disease may also infect dogs and other animals. Its cause is as yet unknown.

Valley fever is endemic to the Lower Sonoran Life Zone which includes the desert areas of California, southern Arizona, Utah, New Mexico, Nevada, western Texas, Mexico, Guatemala, Honduras, Argentina, Paraguay, Venezuela and Colombia. Rodents and dogs in these locations may also contract the disease from the soil.

The fungus grows as mycelium in the soil and propagates during the rainy season. Dry weather and breezy conditions cause the breakup of the mycelium into fragments which are inhaled. It is conjectured that most people who inhabit this life zone will eventually contract the disease which is characterized by flu like symptoms. Many construction workers and archeology students have contracted the disease, since it is frequently found at old American Indian sites due to the presence of charcoal in the soil and other soil charcteristics. Once in the lungs, the mycelial fragments change form into spherules which can spread throughout the body.

None of the diphasic fungi are spread from person to person, and in fact, it is rare for any fungus disease to spread in this manner. One notable exception is ringworm fungi.

Chapter 2
Where Mold Grows

For practical purposes, most of our concerns about mold have been directed toward its growth on indoor structural materials. Common species include *Aspergillus, Penicillium, Cladosporium, Stachybotrys* (Stachy), and *Chaetomium*. The latter two are cellulose-digesting molds that grow on wallboard and its paper backing, carpet backing, and vinyl tile glue-down mastic.

Indoors, they are found growing in clothes dryers that are vented indoors, wet clothes on indoor drying lines, steam from showers and bathtubs, drywall and wood associated with pipe leaks and breaks, overwatering of houseplants in wicker baskets, damp basements or crawl spaces, leaky roofs, backed-up sewers, mud and ice flows, flooding, backed-up drains in air conditioners, refrigerator drip pans and pools of water in the refrigerator, broken or misplaced spiders in evaporative coolers and dirty cooler pads, and a variety of oddities that add water to a home.

Given enough moisture, mold will grow on virtually any substance except for fiberglass, metal, glass, dry porcelain, or dry concrete. It will grow on the paint that is present on these objects, as well as the dust that might be present in them. Otherwise, when liberated from a point source in the home, they will not grow on dry household objects. The caveat here is that the indoor humidity must be kept below 50 to 60 percent. This is difficult in many parts of the country, so a light coating of mold on possessions can be expected, especially in tightly packed closets where no interior light is on to dry the air.

With sufficient moisture, mold will grow on soil, gypsum board, baseboards, carpet backing, carpet pads and tack strips, fabrics, press wood, OSB (oriented strand board), paint and wallpaper, mastics, wood studs, wax on the surface of ceramic or Saltillo tile, dust in fiberglass insulation, and paper products. It will also grow on refrigerator door seals and refrigerator paint; enclosed foods such as cheese and bread, fruits and vegetables, jams and jellies, and meats; indoor and outdoor plants and their soil; beneath the toilet tank lid; and on cotton and leather clothing, belts, and shoes. In nature it has the potential to grow on and spoil virtually every food source. It does not distinguish water damage to structural materials in a hospital from that of a house or an office.

Some mold species release more spores than others. Members of the general group *Aspergillus-Penicillium* release a large number of very small spores into the air under proper conditions of humidity, temperature, and air currents. Others, such as *Stachybotrys, Alternaria, Drechslera,* or *Epicoccum,* release relatively few spores.

In an uncontaminated building, indoor spore counts can vary from less than one hundred per cubic meter of air in the desert southwest to several thousand in more humid parts of the country.

In a contaminated building, the number can increase ten- to thirtyfold or more over their baseline level.

Chapter 3
Climate and Mold

It is not difficult to understand how variations in weather can affect the amount of airborne outdoor mold and its close relatives.

There are two important considerations to keep in mind. First, remember that whatever happens outdoors usually happens indoors, but to a lesser extent and delayed. It occurs through ingress and egress, tracking, and air leakage in the building.

Second, the weather of the day will affect our physical and mental health as our hormone level and sensitivity to environmental circumstances change. See "Weather and Your Health" for a more detailed discussion of this phenomenon.

Now, let's take a closer look at weather and mold.

Rainfall. More rain means more vegetation, the natural food source for mold (and fungi).

Cold. Similar to other life forms, mold has an optimum temperature range for growth and reproduction. It prefers warm and moist to dry and cold.

Hot and dry weather is not friendly to mold reproduction, and air spore counts will decrease significantly when this weather prevails.

Wind causes ground debris to become airborne, and ground debris has mold. Also, the principal method for the spread of infectious and allergenic smuts that attack grains in the Midwest and elsewhere is wind. Finally, wind causes leaves to rub together. This results in the release of the plant epidermis into the air, and this may contain plant pathogens and allergenic species. Wind direction can bring in more mold spores (grain smuts and rusts) and blow out existing spores.

Cold front. A sharp edge to a cold front will stack up airborne particles against it and cause a spike in mold (and particle) counts as it enters a region.

Low barometric pressure signifies that a storm front is incoming. It also means breezy conditions will prevail. These conditions are conducive to the increase in the amount of airborne mold.

High barometric pressure means that stable conditions will prevail, and the amount of mold in the air is likely to remain largely unchanged.

Rainfall directly causes the release of an entire subdivision of fungi when it is struck by raindrops. This is true in the city, the desert, and the forest. These are the sexual phases of common molds. The spores are known as ascospores. The way they are formed is that different strains of the same species of mold conjoin and exchange nuclei. If the strains are 'opposite' they form millions of little packets, each of which has eight spores. (The technical terms are that the strains form ascogenous hyphae through Crozier formation.) This is the sexual phase. Each of the little spores can hit the soil or a plant and grow back into *Aspergillus* or *Penicillium* or into whatever their parents were initially.

Within hours after rainfall, members of these two genera will appear in the air when the sexual forms convert to their asexual forms. In the days immediately following a rainfall, there will be a spike in the number of *Cladosporium, Alternaria,* and other common allergens that are normally present, due in large part to this conversion process. Whether it is the large number of species of ascospores that are present, or the common mold species that many people are familiar with, the number of airborne spores increase prior to (wind), during (water droplet impact) and after (high humidity) a rainfall.

Understanding these conditions is an important part of interpreting mold counts when the indoor environment is sampled. While the number of spores outdoors versus indoors is important, so are the types of spores. If the number of outdoor spores is high they will work their way indoors. If the outdoor count drops off quickly through climate change and one then tests the indoor air, it is possible that the indoor count will be greater than the outdoor count and one might think that there is indoor contamination. However, if the indoor spores are plant pathogens or mushroom spores, or ascospores, then it is unlikely that contamination is present.

Chapter 4

Mold Smell

Our knowledge of chemistry is growing, and now we understand a little more about how the odor of mold is a potential problem. Indeed, the smell of mold can act as a trigger for asthma.

People describe the smell of mold as musty, dirty, and stale. Over twenty volatile organic compounds (VOCs) have been identified with mold growth; however, exposure to VOCs from mold has not been conclusively linked to health effects, especially at the concentrations that have been reported.[1,2] Now we are finding out that in many parts of the country, the odors we thought were due to paints, carpets, and other renovation-related VOCs may be due to the presence of mold.[3,4]

These odors originate from the chemical byproducts of mold growth. If you looked up the names of these byproducts you would find them on the chemical list published by the Occupational Safety and Health Administration (OSHA). These substances include methylene chloride (used as a paint stripper), hexane (paints, adhesives, cleaning fluids), benzene (gasoline), and acetone (nail polish remover), to name just a few of the hundred or more that have been identified. Given this information, it is not difficult to understand why the musty odor we have all encountered can be hazardous to the health of many.

There are a number of factors that affect the production of these VOCs by a given mold. The genus of mold, for instance, makes a big difference. So does the surface the mold is growing on, its food source (wood versus dry wall), and the genetics of the individual mold strain; the strain of *Penicillium notatum* that grows on the cheese in one refrigerator may not produce the same byproducts as that which grows on the cheese in another refrigerator.

Sometimes, the odor of mold can be present without the presence of spores.

If water runs down the wall from a leaky ceiling and behind the wallpaper, then mold growth may occur, although spores will not be able to escape into the air. You can easily check for this by seeing if the wallpaper is bubbling, and then cut a small (half-inch) three-sided flap in the bubble. Peel it back and see if there is mold growth on the wallpaper or on the wall itself. Then close the flap. You can check a number of areas in this manner.

Once you determine the extent of mold growth behind the wallpaper, you are going to have to fix the problem. You can find more detailed instructions in chapter 6, "Case Histories."

In the case of a leaky roof, the attic or crawlspace can become contaminated with mold that is growing on the wood or at the bottom of the insulation. If your air ducts run through this area and there is a small leak in the duct, then the smell of mold, but not the spores, will be pulled into the duct when the unit is turned on. Usually the duct-leak occurs where it attaches to the air-handling unit or joins another section of ductwork. This connection should be examined periodically to ensure that it is tight fitting. In some areas of the country the ductwork is underground. Unfortunately, inspection can be difficult, unless a robot camera is used.

It is beyond the scope of this book to present the various atmospheric conditions that may be present indoors. In general, though, if you live in an area of the country where high humidity and a lot of rain is normal, a leaky home will lead to an increase in humidity indoors, especially in the attic and basement. Condensation will frequently occur there and mold growth will be supported. This mold may infiltrate other areas of the home proper.

Another way for smell to enter the home proper is for fans or a fireplace to create negative air pressure. Attic or basement smells may enter through small openings around recessed (canned) lighting.

Consider the musty odor of mold in the home as a warning sign.

Chapter 5

Toxins from Mold

The subject of mold toxins (mycotoxins) is becoming a regular feature of mold reports and claims made by lawyers.[5] There is as much fiction as there is fact surrounding these chemical substances.

I have served as consultant on a number of lawsuits claiming that fewer than one hundred spores have caused "toxic" injury to a client. A medical doctor who testified in one of these cases stated that he could pinpoint the exact date in years past when his client was exposed to the toxic mold. He never published his findings.

As it grows, mold produces millions, if not billions, of spores. These spores become airborne and are inhaled. (Spores are so small that they remain suspended in the air for a long period of time, as long as there are air currents to keep them aloft.) If there are enough of them, the results can be an allergic reaction. However, under normal circumstances, airborne mold may represent only one part in ten-thousand to one part in one hundred-thousand of 1 percent of the total particle load that we inhale on a daily basis.

As it grows, the mold produces a lot of chemical byproducts. Some of these byproducts have odors because they are chemically lightweight and become airborne very easily. We say that they are volatile, like nail polish remover. Fungal toxins are also byproducts of growth; however, mycotoxins are not considered volatile and are not airborne to any significant extent.

What is the difference between a fungal toxin and an antibiotic? Unlike fungal toxins, antibiotics are more active against bacteria and other fungi than they are against humans and animals. One byproduct of the mold *Penicillium* is penicillin, and it is produced by varying amounts of the same mold that might grow on grapefruit, cheese, or bread. However, *Penicillium* mold can also produce a variety of mycotoxins under the same circumstances.

I have researched published peer-reviewed papers on mycotoxins in the medical literature, crystallized a trichothecene, the major fungal toxin produced by *Stachybotrys* and *Fusarium*, and conducted DNA studies with it. To my regret, experimental mice were also used in the studies.

The subject matter of mycotoxins rivals that of antibiotics,[6] yet may lay claim to more frivolous lawsuits. Similar to asbestos and radon, it is a current health hazard of some merit. Unlike the others, it has the mystique of being biological in origin and, in my opinion, its implications have engendered wholesale concern where none should be present.

Mycotoxins have been discovered in a variety of water-damaged building materials, and in the dust of water-damaged homes. They are not volatile, thus *they are not airborne* as a gas because their molecular weight is fairly large, according to the AIHA.[7] This statement is at odds with other data that are available.[8] In the latter studies cited, direct exposure to fungal toxins induced experimentally through inhalation resulted in various health effects and the toxin was derived from spores that obviously, belonged to a toxic strain of the mold. However, no direct link could be made between the inhalation of spores and a disease state, that could be associated with poisoning in my opinion. I will concede that industrial settings may be different than normal workplace or home contamination issues, because the continual exposure to contaminated grains, for example, may yield symptoms in a select group of persons. Even in those rare cases, the effects of spores alone may not be separated from any toxin they may contain and has little or no relevance to the average homeowner, just as asbestosis among persons who worked with the substance for many years has little relevance to the homeowner.

The presence or absence of specific molds cannot be used to predict mycotoxin presence. Even the presence of the "toxic" mold, *Stachybotrys* (Stachy), that has received so much media attention, does not mean that there are a lot of spores in the air, or that any toxins produced by this mold are present in the wallboard, air, or dust of the home. Much depends on the "strain" of mold that is present, as exemplified by *Penicillium*, mentioned above.

A strain is an identical mold that has been isolated from a different location. In the laboratory, as in nature, ten different strains can be grown. Some may produce no mycotoxin at all, some may produce a little, and some may produce a lot.[9]

As noted above, over the past decade a number of studies have found that Stachy has toxin attached to its spores.[6,10,11] This is a new discovery; prior to that, it was not believed that this could occur. The percentage of homes that have Stachy growing on water-damaged materials may differ in different parts of the country. For example, according to my personal observation of more than six thousand homes, it will grow in 80 to 90 percent of such homes in the desert southwest. The type of building materials used plays a big role in the ability of this mold to grow indoors. The most frequently identified molds found in these instances include members of the small-spored *Aspergillus* and *Penicillium* grouping. Also, expect to find the allergens *Cladosporium*, *Stachybotrys*, *Alternaria* and *Chaetomium* molds. Secondary genera are also found.

Nobody knows how many spores of any mold it takes to make a person ill, or how long one has to inhale them for illness to occur. A lot depends on the state of health of the individual. Infants, the elderly, and those on steroids or chemotherapy are most susceptible because their immune systems are either immature or impaired.

One estimate has it that fourteen million toxic *Stachybotrys* spores per cubic meter of air would have to be inhaled each hour over a twenty-four-hour period for a person to become poisoned. (Personal communication)

Chapter 6
Mold Spore Counts in the Air

It is not surprising that the number of mold spores in the air of cities around the country varies greatly, depending on location and time of the year.

Figures regarding mold (and pollen) data are commonly presented in terms of the number of spores per cubic meter of air.

Regarding the outdoor spore level, the National Allergy Bureau of the American Academy of Allergy and Immunology considers 1 to 6,499 spores per cubic meter as low, 6,500 to 12,999 as moderate, 13,000 to 49,999 as high, and above 50,000 as very high.

In the desert of the San Joaquin Valley (Lower Sonoran Life Zone), the air spore count approaches zero throughout most of the year.

In the desert southwest, the counts average from 100 to 400 for the first six months of the year. This increases to as much as 3,000 during the rainy monsoon season of July and August. Higher concentrations of mold can be found in more vegetated sections of the communities.

Albuquerque, New Mexico, can have a *Cladosporium* count over 20,000 during November.

Des Moines, Iowa, can have a *Cladosporium* count in excess of 27,000 from August through September, with a relatively large number of rust fungal spores in the air. These are plant pathogens associated with grains and grasses.

Areas of Florida, the southeast, and the rainy Pacific Northwest commonly have spore counts of 30,000 throughout much of the year.

In New Orleans, the spore counts outdoors in most flooded neighborhoods tested topped out at 77,000 at one site in Chalmette, and 81,000 at another site in Uptown. *Indoor* spore counts in some flooded homes exceeded 600,000.

The most common type of spores will vary. Usually *Cladosporium* or members of the *Aspergillus-Penicillium* group are the most numerous indoors and outdoors. However, heavily forested areas will have a high proportion of outdoor spores that belong to a variety of mushrooms, such as *Agaricus* and *Coprinus*.

Curiously, I have noticed that there is a great deal of litigation regarding health effects blamed on mold in all the areas mentioned above. This includes areas where the outdoor spore count varies from an average of 400 to an average of 30,000 per cubic meter of air. Lawsuits have been filed against apartment owners who have "allowed" forty spores to be present indoors which, reportedly, adversely affected the health of the occupant.

Chapter 7

Mold Litigation

On occasion, a newspaper story will report on a multimillion dollar settlement awarded in a mold litigation claim, where the plaintiff asked for compensation for damages to property and health.

Most awards of this nature are reversed on appeal. Still, stories about liability issues with mold as the central feature have become a regular part of courtroom life.

Insurance companies were paying tens of millions of dollars on indoor mold contamination due to water damage; now virtually all of them disavow mold damage in their policies, and many will not allow for damage due to water.

What's the difference between water damage and mold occurrence, and why has mold become such a hot issue?

Let's go back to some basics. There are few objects on which mold will not grow, and the areas on which it will grow may surprise the reader.

In recent years, the use of cheaper building materials has led to easier absorption of water and the rapid growth of a wide variety of mold species. A change from plaster walls, on which it is difficult for mold to grow, to gypsum board, on which mold grows readily, is one example.

Glues used in OSB and particle board provide a perfect medium for mold species to proliferate. Include glue-down mastics for tile flooring as another growth medium for mold when flooding occurs.

I have been consulted on a number of lawsuits that claim

that fewer than one hundred spores have caused 'toxic' injury to a client. A medical doctor who testified in one of these cases stated that he could pinpoint the exact date when his client was exposed to the toxic mold, even though the exposure to these hundred spores had occurred years before. He also stated that for forty thousand dollars a year, he could fix the client's mold-related problems, which, without his help, would continue indefinitely. That is his opinion, as he stated on the witness stand.

Even though cause-and-effect health-related issues are hard to prove with mold, the average person on a jury can relate to the purported symptoms.

It's easy to blame mold as the cause of health problems. Something that smells musty, is green or black and fuzzy, is known to cause allergies, and has the mysticism surrounding its production of mycotoxins is a perfect candidate.

To avoid lawsuits, maintain a proactive stance. Take care of water problems when they occur, avoid stalling, and spend the money now rather than later.

Chapter 8

Home Inspection for Mold

The lack of insurance coverage for mold has become commonplace, although several insurance companies will cover the client up to a limit of five thousand dollars.

Homes are like people and cars. They require regular checkups. Here is how to check your home for water damage and mold.

Start the home check at the water sources, and go room by room. Begin with the under-sink areas. Pull out all the contents from the shelves, look for mold on the wall behind the sink, and feel the pipes for leaks. Look at the shelves for warping and staining. Check the upper counter and its possible separation from the walls. Cracks in the caulking are an indication of present or previous water damage.

Refrigerator ice makers are notorious for slow-leak problems and can cause serious water damage. This will occur on the floors and walls, in wall cavities, and beneath kitchen counters.

Pull out the refrigerator and look behind it for water that might be pooling on the floor. If it is, remove the freestanding water and see if you can either tighten the fitting or turn off the water to the ice maker. Sometimes there is a shutoff valve behind the fridge. If there isn't, have one installed.

Examine window ledges for staining and dried up or cracked grout at the edge of the windows. These are usually due to storm damage and suggest that weather stripping may be necessary at that window. Weather stripping is a good idea anyway for purposes of saving energy and keeping out air-borne pollutants.

In the bathroom, look carefully at the shower tiles to ensure that the grout is whole and not cracked. If it is cracked, then odds are that water worked its way behind the tiles. Mold may be present. The good news here is that it will not be airborne. Short of retiling the area, it can be regrouted.

Push on the shower walls. If they are spongy and give, there is a serious water leakage problem.

Water problems in the shower are usually associated with the lower two or more courses of tiles on any side because of grout that is cracked. It is common on the side of the faucet as well.

Also, in the bathroom, look for ceiling stains. Mold commonly grows on ceiling paint. When mold grows on soft paint, it is airborne to a very low extent.

Yeasts and yeast-like forms are more common when there is abundant freestanding water, as in wet walls and counters. This is not considered to be a problem, because airborne yeasts in the home are not linked to respiratory problems. However, if you are very concerned about the presence of mold in the home, then maintaining a dry bathroom would be in order.

Check for ceiling stains in all the rooms. Stains indicate water leakage from above. This frequently occurs at the juncture of additions to the home, at points where a parapet wall meets the roof, and on flat-roof homes, where drain scuppers meet the roof.

Ceiling-related mold can be easily removed by wet-sanding, drying, and repainting. Opening a window or operating the bathroom fan for ventilation is recommended to remove the excessive moisture that results from condensation of hot shower steam.

Frequently, a closet is located on a bedroom wall opposite the bathroom. Pull out the items from the floor of the closet and examine the edge of the carpet. Needle-nose pliers will help you pull up the carpet from the tack strip. Look for water damage on its underside and at the base of the wall. The presence of mold or moisture will tell you that there is a water leak, perhaps from the commode or shower diverter valve, and that water is draining into the wall cavity. If baseboards are present in your home, look for separation of these from the wall, another indication of water.

Sometimes an external water source will cause this same problem. Examples include the presence of an outdoor planter box, a drip irrigation system that waters dirt next to the home, a sprinkler that has gone awry, or rainwater that pools next to an exterior wall. Therefore, include a walk-around of your home as part of the inspection process.

Next, look in the water heater closet for leakage. Check the walls around the base of the heater. Be sure to look behind the heater as best as you can.

If the home has an air conditioner located in a closet, look for water damage where water condensate might not have drained properly. Also check beneath the air return plenum for the presence of mold growth and accumulated dust that might be pulled into the system.

The secret to preventing mold damage in the home is to stop the water damage as soon as possible. A regular inspection will help accomplish this.

Chapter 9

Mold in Apartments

If you live in an apartment, dealing with mold is not a matter of public health; it is a matter of private health. It probably won't be helpful to contact the health department. You will have to work things out with the management.

For decades, apartment renters have fought with the management about moldy units. Water comes from roof leaks, pipe leakages from an upstairs unit, flooding, faulty shower diverter valves, beneath-sink pipe leaks, evaporative coolers, outside sprinklers that water the outside of the buildings, water purifiers, and cracks in the building frame.

In almost all cases, the causative agents are the same as those which contaminate homes. These are called water-marker fungi when they occur indoors. In addition, the number of gram-negative bacteria is known to increase significantly along with the moisture. These produce endotoxins and can lead to flulike symptoms.

The highly allergenic dust mite loves to eat spores in this moist playground.

The airborne concentration of mold spores and bacteria is frequently extremely high under these conditions.

When tenants complain to the management, it's typical for the complaint to go unheeded or for management to stall. After the management inspects the unit and decides that a problem is real, their common cure is a gloss-over. The surfaces of walls are wiped down with chlorine bleach. Unfortunately, the bleach only takes care of the surface contamination. Even worse, it adds moisture to the mold mycelium that has penetrated the walls, aiding its further growth.

Tenants are at a loss. Their recourse is to call a city or county building inspector who may issue a directive for the management to solve the problem. The management then retaliates, evicting the tenant for one reason or another.

If the mold growth becomes intolerable, it may be prudent for the tenants to ask the management for a clean apartment. They may comply with this request, although the tenants will have to pay for the costs of the move under most circumstances. It would be prudent for the tenants to inspect the offered unit before moving into it.

The tenants may sue the management, but the owners and management have attorneys on retainer. In almost every case, tenants lose in court because they don't have an attorney, don't know how to present their case, or don't know what to ask the judge. A cause and effect health issue has to be proven, a letter from a doctor will be required, and the mold will have to be identified to actually be mold and not just discoloration. Many, if not most people make ridiculous health claims and have nothing to back them up. This situation calls for the hiring of a mold expert to evaluate the apartment. Things can get complicated.

If you are a tenant and have a water-damaged unit where mold is widespread, be sure to document your claims with evidence and photographs. Judges need evidence, and pictures are the best kind of documentation as eyewitness accounts will vary, and in these cases will be colored by opinion.

In most cases, the issue revolves around unsightly water damage and mold spots on the wall. In 90 percent of the cases this amounts to almost nothing in terms of health risk. So don't go overboard regarding undocumented health problems or that you or your children *might* have.

The owners of the property may shift their managers to another location so that if a case ever gets to court, they can claim they hired new managers because the others were not efficient. A new cycle of inactivity may begin.

Before a tenant moves into a building, it is important for him or her to ask other tenants about any problems they might have with the neighborhood or the management.

When you take a walk-through, look underneath the sinks for evidence of water leaks. Check the shower stall to ensure the tiles aren't sagging and that the tile grout has been maintained. This is their responsibility. Also, look for stains on the ceiling, water stains on the carpet, and dark areas of mold growth just above the baseboards.

When you discover a problem, notify the management about it, because when you pay rent you are paying for full use of a "healthful" apartment. Anything that develops to lessen the quality of the apartment becomes the responsibility of the management company and the owner of the property. Many states have health and safety laws regarding rental units. These documents are readily available, in most cases, and a copy of them can be obtained by writing appropriate city or county officials or researching them online.

In summary, apartment owners, managers, and tenants all have things to do to ensure the safety of the apartment renter.

Moving out of your apartment in protest of the conditions, regardless of their severity, is breaking the lease, and the management can and will hold you liable for the balance of your lease payments. They will seek this money in court after they have filed suit against you. Working things out is the best solution. However, sometimes your health and that of your children *is* at risk, and that will have to come first.

Chapter 10
Mold in the Office

The relative humidity within an office should be less than 50 percent as measured by a centrally located humidistat. This is because the humidity will be 60 or 70 percent or higher behind pictures or bookcases and other furnishings that are up against the wall. Keeping indoor humidity low is difficult in many areas of the country where outdoor rainfall and high humidity are common.

When the interior air moisture becomes too elevated and a central air-handling system is in place, the humid air will affect the central filter and cause mold growth on that filter. The mold will use the dust as food, and the small-spore allergenic group of universally present *Aspergillus* and *Penicillium* genera will take over. Filters will need to be checked frequently to prevent them from being a point source for mold that is sent into the airspace of the building.

When water from a roof leak penetrates the tile of a dropped ceiling, staining usually occurs. These tiles are inexpensive to replace, and it is a good idea to do so; staining is unsightly, and if enough water is present, *Alternaria* will be there too. *Alternaria* is another universally present and very well studied allergenic mold. The good news is that it is poorly airborne when it grows indoors. The offending tile or tiles should be removed, and the area between the drop ceiling and the roof should be examined as closely as possible to ensure that mold growth is not freely occurring there. If it is, it could present odors over time, and spores might be pulled into the air-handling system.

Mold is usually a nonissue where dry carpets are concerned. Most office carpets are made from low-pile synthetic fabric that offers little or no food source to support mold growth from a water spill, such a tipped-over five-gallon water jug, although it is prudent to clean the spill quickly. This does not include the carpet backing, the pad, or the glue-down mastic, which can support mold growth after prolonged wetness.

Normally it would take a major water intrusion for mold growth to occur in carpeting. Major water intrusions might include a continual ceiling leak or repeated flooding through one of the exterior doors as a result of rainfall or a lawn sprinkler that continually wets one wall. It may be necessary to pull back a wet carpet for inspection of its underside, though the presence of water stains does not mean mold is growing. The dry-out process should be accomplished within two to three days.

Large potted plants in offices are notorious for their destruction of carpeting (and vinyl and ceramic tile) through mold and water damage at their base. The soil may also have mold growth at its surface, and any wicker present can also become contaminated.

The plants should always be placed in a catch basin to ensure that moisture from watering does not wet the carpet. Otherwise one or more mold species will begin to grow and become airborne. This should be done even when the pot is entire and without a drain hole, as the bottom of the pot may be cracked.

It is possible for carpeting to become wet beneath the pot even when a catch basin is present. This may occur if it is close to an external wall where moisture can migrate through the slab from outdoor water sources. For this reason, the pot should be moved occasionally to check the carpet beneath it.

Finally, check the water sources beneath the kitchen and

bathroom sinks and the water supply lines to the commode and the drinking fountain. The refrigerator is frequently problematic in that numerous employees make use of it, and old and moldy food may be present in a back corner or a door shelf. (Please refer to the chapter on Refrigerators.)

Depending on the office and area of the country, other points of interest may include water purification system hookups, water heater, and drip irrigation and sprinkler systems.

Chapter 11

Mold Remediation

Most professional mold remediation companies (MRC) will follow the IICRC S-500 guidelines for professional water damage restoration.[12]

An MRC will endeavor to work quickly and efficiently in order to get their crew to move on to the next job. The last thing they want to do is get delayed at a single location. Delay ties up their equipment, especially when they have a lot of jobs to do. Delay also costs more money for those involved with the project, including the insurance company, and possibly the homeowner. Furthermore, delay inconveniences the residents, who have to deal with a containment barrier at one or more locations, furnishings that have been moved, and the annoying noise of the air scrubbers, which may deprive them of sleep. The more time it takes to resolve the problem, the more these inconveniences will wear on the occupants.

A typical job generally follows a general procedure, as described below.

The homeowners discover a large amount of mold growth on the lower wall of the master closet. To address the problem, they call an MRC out of the phone book or obtain a name by asking around. Alternatively, they might first report the incident to their insurance company, which calls one of the MRC vendors they work with.

The homeowners ask for an estimate. The MRC asks about insurance coverage if an insurance company hasn't referred them.

The MRC comes to the home, where they determine that there is moisture on the wall of the closet and that the moisture is coming from the bathroom on the opposite side of the closet wall. The vanity or commode is probably located on that wall where a pipe leak has occurred.

The MRC may also discover that the carpet in the closet is contaminated and will have to be removed. The homeowners must then decide what to do with the contents of the closet. If there is actual mold growth on certain items such as leather belts and shoes, the items may have to be discarded. If there is no mold growth on the contents, they may be laundered, dry-cleaned, or simply moved to another location until the work is completed.

The MRC then critically contain the bathroom and the closet on the other side. The mold is extensive, which means that there is a strong likelihood that a high concentration of spores has affected the bedroom air, and the bedroom itself will have to be contained at the doorway.

They cover the bathroom doorway and closet entry with heavy-gauge plastic, possibly starting several feet back from the entry to permit working room, The containment can be breached by a zipper or flap opening.

In the bathroom, they'll pull the vanity and inspect the back of it to determine if it can be repaired or if must be replaced. The wall behind the vanity will probably be green or black with mold. They will cut this wall until they do not observe any further mold, then cut another twelve to sixteen inches beyond that. They will cut through the wall on two sides to include the closet side.

The MRC bags and removes contaminated materials from the home. They detail-clean the studs and baseplates and possibly seal them with an approved sealant. Regulations on the proper sealing of structural materials will vary between MRCs and from state to state.

The MRC installs an air filtration machine (air scrubber or negative air machine), which pulls air through a HEPA (high-efficiency particulate air)filter. This will capture any airborne spores that might be present.

As a final step before build-back (reconstruction), a mold expert will be called to conduct an inspection and perform an air test of the remediated area within the containment to ensure that the spore count is sufficiently low to remove the containment. This will be a judgment call.

If the spore count is still elevated, it may be due to a problem with the placement of the air filtration scrubber. It is also possible that the MRC has not discovered all the mold. This is not an uncommon occurrence. If the spore count is still elevated, the mold expert will discuss the matter with the MRC and offer suggestions on how to proceed, at which time the process is repeated.

There are a number of circumstances under which the scrubber will not work well within the containment. This topic is beyond the scope of this book.

Chapter 12

What Is a Disclaimer?

Mold remediation companies often use a disclaimer that frees them from responsibility for the task at hand for various reasons. Here is an example of one. This may be presented for signature to the person who is contracting for the service or presented when the report is given after the work is performed. The former is more frequently used. Although the disclaimer serves as a deterrent, it does not mean that the client cannot file suit for a variety of real or perceived health issues or damages to their property.

Sample Disclaimer

Any recommendations made in this report are just recommendations, and their number and order can and often do vary depending on findings and consultations during the remediation process.

Any data presented in this report are the result of the equipment and techniques employed at the time of the study. Therefore, the opinion expressed by this writer is just an opinion based upon his interpretation of the information at hand and his experience in dealing with similar circumstances. Other persons reading this report may not share these opinions.

Furthermore, any information presented by the contractor relates to his observations and opinions only, which are only valid for the date and time of his visit to the home or facility. The investigator is not responsible for reporting areas of contamination that might exist in portions of the residence or facility that were not inspected or tested.

Any data collected from this home or facility obtained at a future date cannot be construed to be representative of findings obtained at the particular date and time of this study.

Endnotes

1. Mendell, M.J. (1993) Non Specific Symptoms in Office Workers: A Review and Summary of Epidemiological Literature. Indoor Air 3:227-236.

2. Becher, R., et al. 1996. Environmental Chemicals Relevant for Respiratory Hypersensitivity.: The Indoor Environment Toxicology Letters 86:155-162.

3. Wessen, B. and K.O. Schoeps: 1996. Microbial Volatile Compounds–What Substances can be Found in Sick Buildings? *Analyst* 121:1203-1205.

4. Morey, P., et al. (1990) Microbial VOCs in Moisture Damaged Buildings. Healthy Buildings I:245-250.

5. Etzel, R. et al. 1998. Toxic Effects of Indoor Molds. American Academy of Pediatrics. Committee on Environmental Health. April 101:4,712-714.

6. Sorenson, W.G. et al. 1986. Toxicity of Mycotoxins for the Rat Pulmonary Macrophage *in vitro*. *Environmental Health Perspective.* 66:45-53.

7. Field Guide for the Determination of Biological Contaminants in Environmental Samples. A publication of the American Industrial Hygiene Association. 2nd ed. AIHA Fairfax, VA. 2005, p. 173.

8. Bioaerosols. Assessment and Control. American Conference of Governmental Industrial Hygienists (ACGIH) 1999. ACGIH Publ.24.2.2

9. Sorenson, W.G., M.R. Sneller and H.D Larsh. 1975. Qualitative and quantitative assay of Trichothecin: A Mycotoxin Produced by *Trichothecium roseum*. *Appl Microbiol*. 29:653

10. Pasanen, A. et al. 1994. *Stachybotrys atra corda* may produce mycotoxins in respiratory filters in humid environments. Amer Indust Hygiene Assn J. 55:1,62-65

11. Kuhn, D.M. and M.A. Ghannoum. 2003. Indoor Mold, Toxigenic Fungi, and *Stachybotrys chartarum*: Infectious Disease Perspective. Clin Microbiol Rev. American Society for Microbiology.16:1.

12. Institute of Inspection Cleaning and Restoration. 1999. Standard and Reference Guide for Professional Water Damage Restoration. 2nd Ed. IICRC S500. Vancouver, Wash.

The AIHA or American Industrial Hygiene Association, is one of the largest national associations serving the needs of occupational and environmental health professionals practicing industrial hygiene in industrial , government, labor, academic institutions, and independent organizations. Their field book serves as a guide for indoor air sampling that is followed throughout the country by professionals for bacterial and fungal testing procedures.

Section 13

Safe Household Cleaning

I am now offering solutions to our indoor air quality problems. I have addressed the products we buy to eliminate or mask odors and now introduce products that will eliminate the production of VOCs and make our indoor air a lot healthier to breathe.[1]

If we purchase lemons, white distilled vinegar, baking soda, and borax, four inexpensive agents, we have saved hundreds of dollars a year. This is because we will *not* buy dishwashing and laundry detergent (or use a lot less), fabric softener, degreaser, general cleansers and cleaners for floors, tiles, commodes, and countertops, oven and drain cleaners, furniture polish, toothpaste, mouthwash, deodorizers, air fresheners, pesticides, herbicides, and rodent deterrents, antimicrobials and disinfectants, and carpet stain removers.

And that does not count health and beauty aids and cooking aids that will be replaced with the use of these four products. When you make those replacements and do a little research, expect to find hundreds of other tips on saving money and becoming healthier at the same time. Guess what? That means less time spent and lots of dollars saved on doctor visits, and less sick days for the kids. Your pets will be healthier, too.

In this section I present a compendium of information that will transform virtually all household chores into safe and efficient and easily performed tasks. In these days of financial drought, these tips may change a lot of lives. Most of the information has been gleaned from the Internet and brought together for ease of reading. Other materials I gathered from personal experiences and comprehensive books that are on the market.

When I say they are inexpensive, a 76 ounce of 20 Mule Team Borax® costs $4.99 (on line) or approximately one dollar a pound.

Commercially available detergent generally costs over four dollars a pound unless you can get it in bulk or belong to a discount warehouse. Then, it may cost three dollars a pound.

Baking soda also costs from fifty cents to one dollar a pound in bulk.

Vinegar costs approximately $2.39 a gallon.

The cost of lemons varies greatly, but expect to pay .25 to .50 cents each. I priced a 16 ounce bottle of concentrated lemon juice at the local dollar store at $1.50.

Obviously, these prices will vary greatly for a lot of reasons, however, they will be proportionately less than the other supplies that most people purchase regularly.

The cost per bottle of cleaners, cleansers, polishes and pesticides compared with the cost of our famous four products is much greater and the savings are much more. Figure on a one-to-ten ratio is some cases, if not more.

There is not much that is really new here. A lot of what is being presented goes back literally hundred to thousands of years and in modern times, appears daily in a variety of journals, newspapers, books, and other information sources.

Still, I am compelled to pull this information into this volume because it is fitting to do so. It completes the circle and fits into our theme of better air quality.

Each of our four agents has its special qualities, but they also have cross-over attributes. You can use vinegar, baking soda or borax in the toilet bowl, or to clean tiles and sinks, or to freshen up a given area. These products can be used for drain lines or pesticides or for removing stains.

To me, the strength of the lemon is its freshness, its nonchemical scent. Its many uses in foods and beverages are beyond the scope of this book. One drawback? The cost of lemons is going up. Also, dentists tell us that the juice from a raw lemon will destroy the enamel on the teeth. This cannot be replaced. Also, the strong acidity can kill the resident bacteria that inhabit the mouth, thus leading to the formation of canker sores. Adults, and especially children, should be discouraged from biting into the fruit or eating the raw slices. Many asthmatics react to the scent of citrus (and pine). Asthmatics in a household may wish to use alternate methods of housecleaning where the odors (fragrances) of cleaners are not present. This might include the strong smell of acetic acid (vinegar).

Care should be exercised in using a portion (e.g., ½ fresh lemon) in a sachet for air freshening. Green mold usually takes advantage of this fruit, just as it does when the lemon is placed in a baggie in the refrigerator.

I give vinegar the greatest number of points in terms of its versatility and its germ killing power. One drawback is that the light odor of acetic acid can linger in a closed home and may become bothersome if it is used to extreme.

Baking soda's strength is its odor absorbing capabilities.

Hence, I spent more time discussing this compared with its cleaning attributes. The use of baking soda should be limited in terms of its usage in cooking, e.g. tenderizing meat by rubbing it with soda, for persons who are on a low sodium diet.

The real strength of borax and boric acid are their insecticide, pesticide, and antifungal properties in addition to their cleaning power. This is an amazing product. Its drawback is that the powder of boric acid is difficult to apply. Alternatives are offered.

I omitted the traditional cleaning agents of ammonia and chlorine bleach (sodium hypochlorite) for a several reasons. While they are effective when used according to recommendations, most homeowners are already familiar with their uses; they can be harmful and destructive if overused; and, they emit powerful smells that can be respiratory irritants. They are mentioned elsewhere in this volume. The two should *never* be mixed together. To do so would cause the release of poisonous chlorine gas and hydrochloric acid into the air and into the lungs.

I also omitted hydrogen peroxide from our list because, while the traditional 3 percent solution is antibacterial, many of the uses that are touted are unproven and the agent may do more harm than good. For example, its antifungal power is unproven and so are most of its health benefits. It is a bleach and has to be used with care and it breaks down quickly in the presence of oxygen and sunlight. It can be harmful or fatal if ingested and its use as a mouthwash or whitening agent in toothpaste should be limited to prevent damage to the teeth, although its whitening capabilities in this regard are renown.

Disinfecting qualities

In 2000, the Good Housekeeping Institute reported on the

CBS Television program *48 Hours,* that as a disinfectant, a normal 5 percent solution of vinegar will kill 99 percent of bacteria, 82 percent of mold, and 80 percent of viruses. They reported that vinegar will be effective on countertops where *Staphylococcus Streptococcus, E. coli, Salmonella,* viruses, and other disease causing agents can be found, as well as on refrigerator and microwave handles. Because it is not registered as a disinfectant with the EPA and claims regarding its disinfecting qualities are not widely known, only word-of-mouth spreads the information.

We can have inexpensive alternatives to pressurized and scented pesticides, floor and furniture polishes that contain VOCs and serve as respiratory irritants and carcinogens, and alternatives to cleaning agents that are fragranced with an endless stream of scents. A list of cooking tips will not be provided and I will concentrate on those tips that serve to steer us away from hazardous chemicals.

When I mention pesticides, I must note that vinegar and borax may be very effective against fungi, bacteria, viruses and other microbial and insect types, but they are not registered as pesticides. Therefore, they cannot claim to be bactericidal, or fungicidal or any one of the two dozen classes of pesticides that are recognized by the government. (Bleach was issued an exemption during the 2001 contamination of various governmental offices by the anthrax bacillus.)

When trying these different uses for the first time, the reader should use them on inconspicuous areas first, to test the mixture on the material that it is being applied to. For example, if vinegar is to be used to remove a carpet stain, first ensure that the color of the carpet will not be compromised by trying the mixture on a small area in a closet.

There are literally hundreds of uses for each of the products mentioned in this section and unfortunately, only a few examples are presented. On the upside, salient references are given so that the reader can pursue the topic further.

Some websites, such as that of The Vinegar Institute, only serve as a catch all for suggestions and recommendations, and do not endorse those suggestions. However, I have had great success using many of these tips in my own household in terms of cleaning grease from the stovetop and microwave interior, sanitizing counter tops and refrigerator and microwave doors, as well as for the cleaning of tile floors and removing stains from carpeting. I have used these products in my shower and commode. I have used them as pesticides and to remove odors from carpeting.

The best part is that I avoided the purchase of products that are overly fragranced and which contain petroleum distillates. Thus, my family's health was not compromised.

Chapter 1

Use a Lemon for Many Nontoxic Cleaning Chores

There are many safe uses for the lemon for the average household, as long as overuse is not presented and an asthmatic person is not present.

Musgrove presents 15 uses of lemons[2] and others present information regarding cleaning with lemon juice.[3,4] These are only two of hundreds of references that pertain to this topic.

If the reader is fortunate enough to obtain a good supply of lemons, it is recommended that you squeeze out the juice into a glass container and place it in the freezer. Freeze the rinds in a plastic bag for later use in freshening the garbage disposal. Then freeze a supply of whole lemons and keep a few for your immediate usage.

As an alternative to whole lemons, concentrated lemon juice is readily available in the market. It's inexpensive and doesn't take up storage space.

Note: 6 medium size lemons = 1 cup of juice and 1 medium lemon = 3 teaspoons of juice

Hair Bleaching and Highlighting: As an alternative to harsh and toxic chemicals that are used in commercial products that make your hair brittle and may affect your breathing, try this: If you want to lighten your hair, mix ¼ cup lemon juice with ¾ cup water and rub it into your hair. Repeat as necessary. Individual experimentation will be required to ascertain the level of color desired.

Fingernails: To bleach and harden nails and to avoid chemical treatments (acetone---a respiratory irritant) for removal of polish, rub a portion of the squeezed lemon over the nails after the juice has been extracted to be saved, or used elsewhere.

Cleaning Tupperware: To avoid the use of strong chlorine bleach, squeeze some lemon juice into the container from a lemon slice or a half and add some baking soda. Use the lemon rind to bleach out the stains. (Disinfection should not be a problem at this point.)

Shower doors, tiles, and other glassware: Water stains remain after washing because of lime deposits from hard water. These can be dissolved by the acid in the lemon. A dilute solution of warm lemon juice will quickly clean water drops from bathtubs, doors, and fixtures. Use half to a full lemon squeezed into a quart of warm water. A sponge dipped in the juice will suffice to remove the scum. Then dry. Some people use vinegar to do the same job, although it lacks the natural lemon scent.

Faucets: Rub them with a lemon peel, then wash and dry them with a soft cloth to shine and remove the spots. This natural method of cleaning has disinfectant qualities.

Kitchen: Wipe both sides of the grater with a lemon to loosen attached cheese or vegetables and other foods. (The grater should be plastic to avoid oxidizing any metals.)

Microwave: Boil 1 cup water and 4 tablespoons lemon juice. Boil for 5 minutes and clean the unit with ease.

Cooking: At the risk of getting too far afield, it is important for me to give you this information: If you are reducing your sodium or fat intake, you can cut back significantly on your salad dressing and add a little lemon onto your salad. You can also accomplish the same goal by adding a little lemon juice to your steamed vegetables, soups and stews and either eliminate or reduce the salt that you would otherwise add to the dish.

Odors: A half lemon placed on the shelf of the refrigerator will absorb odors.

Tubs and sinks: To avoid the use of bleach and heavy cleaners, rub the areas with half a lemon dipped in borax. The lemon will remove the lime buildup and the borax will remove the soap and grease.

Copper and brass polish: Use the juice undiluted, or mix with it table salt to make a paste. Rub, wash with distilled water to avoid spotting, and dry.

Furniture polish: Mix one part lemon juice with one part olive oil or vegetable oil. You may need to increase the amount of oil to your preference. The furniture is left with a fine gloss with no outgassing from the petroleum distillates commonly used in commercial polishes.

*Evaporative coolers:*Use lemon juice as a descaler.

Paintbrushes: Dip the hardened brushes into boiling lemon juice. Lower the heat immediately. (Boil the juice first, then move the pot to the outdoors.) Leave the brush in the pot for fifteen minutes and then wash it in soapy water.

Paint: A few drops of lemon juice in outdoor house paint will keep insects away while you are painting.

Paint on glass: Apply hot lemon juice to the paint with a soft cloth or soft tissue. Leave it on until it is nearly dry, then wipe off the old paint.

Garbage disposal:. Toss used lemons into your garbage disposal to keep it clean and fresh smelling.

There are scores of other applications of the lemon. Many of them apply to canning, keeping fruits and vegetables from turning color, maintaining the freshness and color of guacamole when it is exposed to the air, removing blemishes, dishwashing, and for cosmetic purposes.

Chapter 2

Uses of Vinegar

Vinegar is made from the fermentation of ethanol and it is comprised of about 5 percent acetic acid, although higher concentrations (up to 18 percent) may be used for pickling. At this higher concentration, care should be taken because the vinegar can be corrosive and acts as a skin irritant. Its disinfecting qualities were discussed in the introduction to this section.[5-9]

Vinegar can be used as a degreaser when it is combined with baking soda or ammonia. (1 gallon of hot water, one cup household ammonia, ½ cup vinegar, ¼ cup baking soda.)

White distilled vinegar (WDV), red wine vinegar, cider, balsamic, and malt vinegar are five types of vinegar. Most cleaning of the household involves the use of the first and the others are primarily used for food preparation. Brown (cider) vinegar may stain porous materials.

The reader is encouraged to look up Vinegar in Wikipedia, the online encyclopedia, to get a broad description of the types of vinegar that are available, how they are made and how they are used.

Caution: Never use vinegar on marble.

Use as a fabric softener: Because it cuts detergent residue, WDV vinegar makes a great fabric softener substitute for families with sensitive skin. Add some vinegar to a rag or bath towel and throw it into the dryer with clothes (1/2 cup).

Use as a disinfectant: Counter surfaces may be treated with

WDV as an antibacterial agent. It is not useful as such when taken internally.

Garbage disposal cleaner: Fill an ice tray with one cup WDV and enough water to finish the tray. Place in the freezer and use the cubes to grind in the disposal. Then flush it with cold water.

Clean and disinfect wood cutting boards: Wipe with full strength WDV.

Coffee maker cleaner: Fill the reservoir with WDV and run it through a brewing cycle. Rinse thoroughly with water when the cycle is finished. (Check the owner's manual for specific instructions.)

Evaporative coolers: Add a quart to the water reservoir to dissolver lime in the pads and to disinfect the unit.

Brass and copper polish: Dissolve 1 teaspoon of salt in 1 cup of WDV and stir in flour until it becomes a paste. Apply paste to the metals and let it stand for about 15 minutes Rinse with clear warm water and polish until dry.

Clean the microwave: Boil a solution of ¼ cup WDV and 1 cup of water in the microwave and let stand for several minutes. The vapors will loosen splattered-on food particles.

Clean the refrigerator: Wash with a solution of equal parts water and WDV.

Remove refrigerator smells: (First, check the unit for old fruits and vegetables and discard them.) Place 1 cup apple cider vinegar in a glass and set in refrigerator. This will remove any odor within 2 days.

Cleaner dishes and glasses. Pour 1 ½ cup to 2 cups of WDV in the bottom of the dishwasher, along with regular dishwasher soap. Wash full cycle.

Grease cutter: Add a few tablespoons to WDV to your dishwashing soap. Use a washcloth with vinegar to clean greasy kitchen walls.

Bathtub film: Remove by wiping with WDV and then with baking soda. Rinse clean with water.

Shower doors and surround: Rub down doors and tiles with a sponged soaked in WDV to remove soap residue.

Toilet bowl cleaner: Add 3 cups of WDV to bowl and let it stand for a half-hour. Brush then flush.

Unclogging the showerhead: Soak a terry cloth towel in WDV and wrap it around the shower head overnight to dissolve the lime.

Unclog a drain: Pour one cup of baking soda down your drain followed by one cup of vinegar. They will interact. After a few minutes, turn on the hot water and flush out the clog. (The acidic vinegar will combine with the sodium bicarbonate to create sodium acetate and carbonic acid. The latter decomposes into water and carbon dioxide.)

Kill grass and weeds: Pour full strength WDV directly on driveway and sidewalk grass and weeds.

Paintbrush softener: Soak the paintbrush in hot WDV, and then wash out with warm, sudsy water.

Furniture polish: Mix olive oil and WDV in a one-to-one ratio and polish with a soft cloth. Experiment on area of the furniture that is not conspicuous to ascertain the effective of this ratio—it may need to be adjusted, e.g., you might want to increase the amount of olive oil.

Clean fireplace doors: Use an equal mixture of WDV and water, spray on, and wipe off.

Wine stains: Spots caused by wine can be removed from 100 percent cotton, cotton polyester and permanent press fabrics if done so within 24 hours. Sponge WDV directly onto the stain and rub away the spots. Then clean according to the directions on manufacturer's care tag.

Wash and freshen clothes: Add 1 cup WDV to the last rinse cycle to dissolve alkalies in soaps and detergents and will soften cotton and wool blankets.

Lint: Keep lint from clinging to your dark clothes by adding ½ cup vinegar to the rinse cycle.

Bee sting: Pain can be lessened by soaking the area in vinegar.

Stop itching: Apply a paste from WDV and cornstarch (body talc). Keep on until itch disappears.

Soothe a sore throat: Add a teaspoon of WDV in a glass of water, gargle, then swallow.

On ceramic tiles: Use ¼ cup vinegar to one gallon warm water. Use a toothbrush in full strength vinegar and gently scrub tough spots in the grout between the tiles.

Discourage puppies: If puppy still returns to a same place in the carpet to do his duty, spray the area with vinegar to turn him away.

Chapter 3
Uses of Baking Soda

Baking soda, or sodium bicarbonate, is related to washing soda, or sodium carbonate. The North American supply of baking soda comes from the state of Wyoming.[10] It is found dissolved in many mineral springs and other aqueous areas. It is deep mined and recovered as both sodium bicarbonate and sodium carbonate (washing soda). The former has more carbon dioxide attached to the molecule which is released during the cooking process. Soda has many important functions, in part because is has properties of both an acid and a base. In the body, it occurs naturally and serves as a buffer to ensure the stable pH of the blood. Its uses in cooking are not applicable to our discussion of a safer and more chemical-free environment.

Information regarding the uses of baking soda is amply available.[11-16]

Some experts suggest the following concentrations of baking soda for various uses: For a solution, 4 tablespoons of soda in 1 quart of warm water; for a paste, 3 parts soda and one part water (mix); to sponge, soda applied lightly to a clean damp sponge; or sprinkle directly onto a surface. According to Arm & Hammer®, in non baking uses you don't need to worry about using too much baking soda.[17]

Absorb Odors: Use a tray of soda in the refrigerator. It can be sprinkled liberally on a carpet and allowed to stand for several hours before vacuuming. It can be applied to shoes and socks to remove odors. It can be added to the bottom of old discarded panty hose by filling the toe or foot portion, cutting and tying it off to create a cheap, safe and effective absorbent device for the home, laundry basket, kids room, and car. With the use of 1-2 cups soda in a bucket of warm water, the walls of the home can be washed to remove household smells, including tobacco odors. This is a good technique to use if you are putting up the house for sale or moving into another home. It can also be sprinkled on the bottom of crisper bins and covered with a paper towel to keep down odors. Soda will absorb the odors from animal urine, pastrami, ammonia, gasoline and oil and many others. Smelly clothing can be placed in a plastic bag with lots of soda and kept overnight before washing. Then add one cup soda to the rinse cycle. Wash garbage cans and baby diapers with soda. Cover the bottom of a clean kitty litter box with 1 part soda and add 3 parts litter over it. To remove strong odor from your hands, wet them and rub vigorously with soda.

It is advised that the use of baking soda as an antacid be reconsidered. This is not because it doesn't work, but because there are many variables that relate to personal habits and medical cautions. If you are going to purchase a product promoted as an antacid, be sure to read the label or consult with your physician.

Toothpaste and Deodorant: These commercial products are available that have soda in them. Make a paste with water. The paste can also be used wet or dry in this mode as a deodorant. Or, you can just sprinkle soda on your wet toothbrush and use it immediately.

Clean Car Battery Terminals: Remove acid buildup on terminals and cables by dissolving a couple of tablespoons of soda in warm water and pouring the solution onto the affected area to neutralize the acid.

Insect Bites: Make a paste of three parts soda to one part water to relieve insect bites.

Extinguish Small Fires: Keep a box of soda handy in the

kitchen to apply to small stovetop fires or electrical fires. Apply by the handful. It is also said to put out fires in clothing, fuel, wood, upholstery and rugs. It must not be poured into fires within deep fryers as the grease will splatter.

Washing clothes: Add to the rinse cycle to serve as a water softener and to remove odors.

Pesticide and herbicide: The high concentration of sodium in the bicarbonate is harmful to insects, but not to plants. Use a couple of tablespoons in your plant sprayer.

Clean combs and brushes with soda to remove grease and odors.

Scour marble, Formica, and plastic surfaces with a paste of soda and water.

Burned pots and pans: Pour soda over the bottom and moisten with water. Allow to stand overnight before scouring.

Relieve sunburn and bee stings: Make a paste of soda and water and apply until pains lessen.

Renew: Soak old sponges, nylon scrubbers and scrub brushes by soaking them overnight in a solution of 4 tablespoons baking soda to 1 quart of water.

Plastic storage containers: Scrub the container with a paste of lemon juice and baking soda.

Erase crayon pencil, ink, and furniture scuffs from painted surfaces. Sprinkle soda on a damp sponge, rub clean, and rinse.

Chapter 4

Uses of Borax

———

Boron is an element and is found naturally in combination with sodium, calcium, magnesium, and oxygen. In this state the mixture is called a borate.

Borax, or sodium tetraborate, is mined from the soil in this complex and is usually a white powder consisting of soft colorless crystals that dissolve easily in water.

Boric acid is a crystalline material derived from borax.

Technically, borax is not considered acutely toxic, but still should not be ingested or used around food.

Commercially sold borax is popularly sold as 20 Mule Team Borax.® Its many uses include its wide-ranging insecticidal applications. It is also antifungal and can be used as a fire retardant.

It does not contain phosphates or chlorine and will not harm washing machines, corrode pipes, or adversely affect septic tanks.

(This product has not been tested or received approval from the EPA for use as a "27 pesticide.")[18]

Insecticide: Borax is used to kill ants, roaches, fleas, lice, silverfish, termites, spiders and weeds. It acts as a stomach poison when ingested by insects.

Olkowski and coauthors recommend boric acid, rather than borax, for pest control as the major tool within an integrated program against roaches.[19,20,21] However, when it is used as a powder, it is less safe and it is inconvenient to work with. Look for brands such as Roach Prufe® made by Copper Brite, and

Roach Kill® made by R-Value that contain an anti-caking compound to resist moisture. Some brands even have an electrical charge that helps the powder adhere to the insect's body. With roaches, expect to see a lag time of five to ten days before the pests begin to die.

Boric acid baits contain a pest formulation that includes an attractant. The paste can be applied to cracks and crevices and is particularly useful in very moist areas.

Similar to vinegar, borax has not been approved as a traditional pesticide by the EPA. One reason for this is that it is a naturally occurring substance.

Rodent deterrent: In areas where rodents have been spotted, sprinkle borax along the perimeters of the rooms where the floors meet the walls. Rodents will avoid these areas. The borax strip will also keep insects from entering the home.

Humidifiers: To remove microbes and odors, dissolve one tablespoon of borax per gallon of water before adding to the unit and allow it to stand for one to two hours. Wipe down the unit, pour out the solution, and rinse before adding fresh water. Repeat every three to six months or as needed.

Candle Making: Reduce ash and smoke by dissolving 1 tablespoon table salt and 2 tablespoons borax in one cup of warm water. Soak heavy twine (wick) for at least 24 hours and allow it to thoroughly dry before using.

Laundry Booster: Borax acts as a water conditioner boosting the cleaning power of detergent by controlling alkalinity. By doing so, the detergent can effectively attach to dirt and odor-causing chemicals in the clothing. This serves to deodorize them and aids in the removal of stains and soil

Garbage and Laundry Pails and Barrels: Wash out with a solution of borax and water (approximately half cup per five gallons).

Dishwasher: Save on dishwasher detergent. Mix a supply of an equal amount of borax and baking soda and put it in the soap dispenser of the unit.

Carpet treatment: Borax can remove stains from a carpet if you mix it into a paste and rub it into the stain. Let the paste dry and vacuum it away; and to make the carpet smell fresh spray it with a fine mist of water and sprinkle on borax. Vacuum after it dries.

Endnotes:

1. *Homemade Cleaning Products*:www.Home Improvement: DIY Network

2. Musgrove, R. *The 15 Secret Uses of Lemons.* www.Lifescript.com.

3. Cobb, L. *Cleaning with Lemon Juice.*
www.housekeeping.about.com/od/environment/a/lemonscleaning.htm

4. Sheldon, J. *Lemons are Not Just for Lemonade: 31 Uses for Lemons and Lemon www.gomestic*.com/Homemaking/Lemons-are-Not-Just-for-Lemonade.5200...

5. Henderson, C. *How to Use Vinegar to Clean.*
http://www.ehow.com/how_4892540_use-vinegar-clean.html

6. Harold, CM. *How to use Vinegar to Clean.*
Natural Healthy Home Cleaning Tips - Vinegar and Baking Soda Cleaning Recipes. http://www.eHow.com/how_4723922_use-vinegar-clean.html

7. Michael, P. 254 *Uses for Vinegar and Counting.* www.wisebread.com/254-uses-for-*vinegar*-and-counting

8. *Uses and Tips.* The Vinegar Institute www.versatilevinegar.org

9. Hancock, S. The *Many Uses of Vinegar.* www.Lifescript.com

10. Lansky, V. 1995. *Baking Soda. Over 500 Fabulous Fun and Frugal Uses You've Probably Never Thought Of.* Book Peddlers.

11. Hardage, R. *10 New Uses for Baking Soda.* www.realsimple.com/realsimple/content/0,21770,1030037,00.html

12. 22 *Effective Baking Soda Uses.The Latest Home Advice!* www.living.aol.com/baking-soda-uses

13. *101 Uses for Baking Soda.* www.apartmenttherapy.com/ny/cleaning/101-uses-for-baking-soda-056.

14. *HowStuffWorks Uses for Baking Soda: Guidelines for Health and Beauty.* howstuffworks.com/uses-for-baking-soda-health-and-beauty-ga.htm.

15. *Sixty Uses of Baking Soda*. www.thefarm.org/charities/i4at/lib2/60soda.htm.

16. Sodium bicarbonate uses. www.RightHealth.com/KidneyInfection

17. www. Arm and Hammer

18 *Borax: The Twenty Mule Team.;* Published by U.S. Borax Inc.; Undated (1980s-'90s). www.scvhistory.com/scvhistory/borax-20muleteam. htm ·

19. Olkowski, W., S. Daar, and H.Olkowski, 1993. *Common-Sense Pest Control. Least Toxic Solutions for Your Home, Garden, Pets and Community.* Taunton Press, Newtown. P. 226.

20. Tritten, L. *The Many Uses of Borax.* Home » Categories » Home Life » Consumer Information » searchwarp.com/swa277269.htm. The Many Household Uses of Borax. homeparents.about.com/cs/householdtips/a/borax.htm.

21. *How to Use Borax Around the House.* How to Kill Fleas With Borax. http://www.ehow.com/how_2123273_use-borax-around-house.html

Section 14

Other Valuable Information

In this section we will present information to the reader that is rarely encountered elsewhere.

In this section, I present pollen and mold data from around the country so that, if you are planning a visit to one of the cities listed, you will know what to expect and when to expect it.

I discuss in some detail the fascinating subject of how weather affects our health. Some of our problems may not be reactions to foods or chemicals; it may just be a due to a change in the weather. Discover why this is.

You will find out about the microbes in our environment; and you will learn the real meaning of the term synergism and how it may contribute to our worsening health, given our exposure to indoor pollutants and to the weather of the day.

Be prepared to read about my belief that television is an asthma trigger. It's a concept that makes sense to me; let's see if it makes sense to you.

Chapter 1
Aerosol Sprays

The first aerosol patent was issued in 1899, but aerosol containers didn't come into use until 1940, when insecticides were packaged. Now they are sold in aerosol cans by the tens of millions each year. Aerosol containers are used for hairsprays, deodorants, and hundreds of home and personal care products.

The main problem with aerosol sprays is the general broadcast of their pressurized stream and their toxic ingredients. Hairsprays, for instant, contain shellac, plasticizer, silicone, lanolin, perfume, vegetable gums, and a variety of alcohols.

When the fine spray is broadcast, the liquid particles are readily airborne and spread throughout the household, to be inhaled by other adults, children and pets. Once inhaled by the respiratory tract, their ingredients are absorbed into the lungs. These micro-droplets are visible under a microscope, when air testing of a home (or school) is conducted. They measure just a few microns in size, well within the PM-10 respirable range.

The pump sprayer poses fewer respiratory problems than do the pressurized aerosols. The droplets are much larger. As such, they are not inhaled into the deeper lung spaces, do not travel far in the airways of the home, and do not require a propellant.

Pump sprayers are generally less expensive than aerosol canisters and last much longer.

Chapter 2

Weather and Your Health

Bioclimatology is the study of the effects of climate and living organisms. For the purposes of this discussion, a more accurate term would be bioweatherology, or the study of how weather affects our health. Climate refers to the long-term condition of a region or the planet as a whole—an average of daily weather statistics—while weather refers to daily changes in atmospheric conditions.

There are five basic components to weather: temperature (usually measured at ground level), prevailing wind, humidity, barometric pressure, and cloudiness, all of which affect our well-being.

The study of weather and health can be traced back thousands of years to almost every society on Earth, from the ancient Chinese to Persians, Europeans, Scandinavians, and Latin Americans. Hippocrates expounded on the subject. Today, ample literature is available to describe virtually every climatic condition and its effect (purported) on the human. Many of the claims are solidly backed with facts, others are pure speculation, and still others are backed only by contradictory evidence.

The human body is dynamic and it changes by the year, season, day, and minute. We operate on circadian rhythms; our hormone levels change throughout the day, along with our sleep patterns and nutritional supply. External factors affect us all the time, and sunlight and weather patterns are no exception.

Indeed, the subject is so popular and useful that Scandinavian peoples are known for their regular broadcasts on the topic based on the weather of the day.

Many thousands of books and hundreds of thousands of pages have been written on this subject. In terms of how it applies to this book on indoor air quality, it is all inclusive. One basic rule of thumb is that whatever happens outdoors usually happens indoors, but to a lesser degree, and frequently with a delayed effect. In short, there is no escape.

The good news is that sometimes we can blame our sluggishness or our poor attitudes and behavior on the weather.

Let's take a brief look at what this subject matter is all about. Key terms include serotonin, ions, cloudy, rainy, incoming storm, sunshine, drop in barometric pressure, cold, colors, heat, high and low relative humidity, hot and cold winds, strong or weak storm front, general heat, and general cold.

Obviously, sunshine can burn us and cause skin cancer, while extreme cold can cause frostbite and extreme heat can cause dehydration.[1]

Our intent here is to explore how many of these climatological (weather) conditions affect most of us in ways other than the obvious and in terms of our daily physical and mental health and well-being.

Barometric pressure

Let's start with one of the most basic concepts: a drop in barometric pressure due to an incoming storm front. The main clinical symptoms are headaches and joint aches. Those persons with arthritis of various types are particularly affected. Other common symptoms include malaise (weakness and not feeling up to par) and behavioral changes for the worse. The latter has been noted for children.

A reduction in barometric pressure, especially a sharp reduction, causes an influx of tissue fluid into areas where previous scar tissue has formed, as well as areas where there were previous injuries. This influx of fluid from blood vessels and surrounding tissues causes them to swell and press on nerve endings, with pain as the result. These areas most commonly include knuckles of the hands, lower back, shoulders, and places where virtually any scar tissue or previous breaks have formed.

Headaches occur during drops in barometric pressure because the meninges swell. Meninges are the three membranes that cover the brain and spinal cord—the central nervous system.

Those who are prone to headaches might do well to plot them on a calendar and correlate their occurrence with storm fronts. Begin plotting two days before the event and continue until two days after the event. This is the normal time span for headaches to begin and end, depending on the severity of the event.

The sharpness of the drop in barometric pressure is frequently a measure of the severity of the swelling and the pain. Watch the weather reports for incoming storm fronts and obtain an inexpensive barometer to personally monitor the weather.

If the reader is contemplating taking an anti-inflammatory medication such as aspirin or ibuprophen to lessen their symptoms before, during, and after a weather-related incident, they are advised to consult with their doctor first.

Weather can affect gout

Gout is a form of arthritis. The painful condition is caused by the presence of uric acid crystals in the joints. Specifically, when certain rich foods are taken in excess, the kidneys are unable to filter out the excessive amount of purines and pyrimidines. The result of this is that uric acid crystals are formed. A few noteworthy examples of rich foods include shellfish, alcohols in general,. including red wine in particular, organ foods (kidney, liver, and tongue), corn beef, and pastrami.

Frequently, hands and feet are affected when tissue fluid infiltrates those extremities due to the crystalline presence. Often, only one or two joints are affected, although the entire ankle and foot can swell to a great extent. The pain is frequently severe and can last for several days, weeks, or even a lifetime, if the diet is not changed. (Medications such as Allopurinol are available to prevent the formation of uric acid crystals.)

Gout has been called the Benjamin Franklin disease because of his years-long affliction. It is a form of arthritis; and as such, weather will cause the swelling of arthritic joints that are susceptible to gout. If you are prone to this affliction, you might keep track of your diet and log the rich foods you ate the day before or so before your attack.

Keeping track of our diet is crucial to our understanding of our daily afflictions. There are numerous factors that can affect our joint aches. In addition to the weather of the day, these include the ingestion of monosodium glutamate (msg), alcoholic beverages, especially red wine, sports activities, viruses, eating of rich foods such as animal organs including tongue, kidneys, livers, and brains, heredity, and, as always, the unknown.

Environmental changes

Going from a dark interior to bright sunlight can trigger a round of sneezing. This is called vasomotor rhinitis and is actually an automatic reaction rather than an affliction.

Going from an air-conditioned interior to hot bright sunlight can lead to a headache. The reverse is also true.

In the morning, the air of a room rotates in a clockwise manner; it goes in the opposite direction during the cooler evening hours. This natural air movement will create more airborne dust and may trigger a sneezing attack.

Wind

Behavioral changes are common among children, adults and pets when windy conditions prevail. More traffic accidents occur, more people wake up nervous and stay that way for hours to days, and acting out becomes more commonplace. There are a lot of factors that interact here. One factor is serotonin.

Serotonin is a neurotransmitter produced by the pineal gland of the brain. It plays a major role in the regulation of mood, sleep, sexuality and appetite. Changing levels of serotonin have been measured for decades as the weather changes and can result in depression, aggressive behavior and anxiety disorders. It is found in the brain, blood and various tissues of the body where it also stimulates the smooth muscles of blood vessels to constrict.

Some investigators believed that positive ions were at fault, while others could not find a correlation between behavior and ion changes in the air.

Theories state that hot winds blow along sand, while cold winds blow down icy mountain slopes. Each brings about an increase in serotonin production. This is because high winds cause the generation of positive and negative ions due to the friction generated between the air and the surface. The ions are asserted to move ahead of the storm front through some mechanism, thus affecting the sensitive person prior to the actual front reaching them. This theory led to the sales of the negative ion generator and is still conjectural. Most serious investigators, however, do not propose that patients should buy a negative ion generator, despite claims by manufacturers. The reader may wish to fully research this matter before purchasing such equipment.

The interested reader may wish to consult the compilation of data presented by Rosen.

Weather conditions that affect the respiratory tract

It is important to note that there are a number of chemical mechanisms whereby the sensitivity of the respiratory tract is affected prior to and during changing climatic conditions.

Examples of direct effects include blowing dust and pollen. Dust storms are not uncommon in many parts of the country. Whatever happens outside also happens inside, but to a lesser extent. In my experience, the outdoor dust level in the PM10 range may increase one hundred-fold or more during a dust storm and the indoor level will increase by ten-fold or more. Obviously, working outdoors and exercising outdoors is not advised during these conditions. Indoors, respiratory health may also falter and unfortunately, all but the best air filters will be unable to reduce the dust particles to any extent where clinical change is noticed.

Also, the leading edge of a storm front can be very cold. This cold air is denser than the warmer air as it moves along, and the edge can be very sharp. Thus, airborne particles back up against it and the concentration of the particles increases tremendously, so that at the point when it reaches us, there is a spike in the concentration of all manner of particulates.

Weather conditions that affect allergies and allergens

Changes in weather can bring about increased sensitivity to allergens. Furthermore, there are several allergens that are affected by weather.

An increase in humidity outdoors generally results in an increase of allergens indoors. This will lead to an increase in the dust mite and mold population. Areas of the home that have the highest humidity include, but are not limited to, the basement, attic, wall cavities, bathrooms, laundry room, rooms at floor level, and walls behind pictures, bookcases, and sofas where air cannot move freely.

The presence of sunlight affects the aerodynamic nature of pollen grains. They are released from the flower more readily in higher numbers and travel on air currents more readily.

Climates that are hot and dry may directly aggravate asthmatic conditions. Cold weather may precipitate an asthma attack, while moisture in the air will assist asthmatics.

Because 85 percent of asthma is allergic asthma, it follows that there are a number of ways climate can affect these millions of people, both directly and indirectly.

Weather sensitivity and gender differences

Three times as many women are weather sensitive as men. In addition, women are more sensitive to small changes.[2,3] Headaches and nervousness are among the most common complaints, along with joint aches.

Other indirect effects of weather on health

Many of Man's illnesses are transmitted by certain vectors, vectors for which the weather conditions must be right to allow their survival or even, occasionally, become benign and bring about epidemic outbreaks.[4] Malaria is one example where the insect vector needs warm temperatures within a certain range and enough moisture in which to lay its eggs.

Chapter 3
Is Television an Asthma Trigger?

There are basically three schools of thought regarding television-viewing practices. Some advocate not watching TV at all. Some advocate watching in moderation and with careful selectivity. And some watch with abandon for lengthy periods of time.

This essay seeks to condemn television. With an understanding of the negative aspects of TV watching, viewers may back off the hours spent in front of the screen. This is a good thing.

The average American watches three to five hours of TV per day, seven days a week. Most references report that children spend nearly three hours a day watching TV and more time on the computer, for a total of twenty-eight hours per week as a minimum figure.[5] Over the period of a year the total comes to 1,456 hours.

I do not disparage the use of television by the elderly or the infirm, who hang onto its noise and images as they would hold onto a dear friend in time of need. However, young, healthy people who have the ability to do other things should consider that the 1,456 hours we lose to TV computes to 182 eight-hour days: enough time to learn several new languages, learn a completely new trade, write a novel, read the complete works of Shakespeare or Josephus, learn the fundamentals of rocket science or ornithology, or study ten college courses. That's per person per year.

I have always found it interesting that we complain about

incompetent teachers, while both parents and their children languish in front of the television.

Television eats up our free time so we have less time to spend with the family, eat a decent meal, go on vacation, exercise, or earn extra income.

By the time he or she is sixty-five years of age, an average American will have viewed two million commercials and will have spent *nine years* of life staring at artificial light and ever-changing images, like a never-ending talking slide show.

Americans are not unusual in their viewing habits. These figures are actually lower than in many countries.

TV is an addiction of both the rich and the poor. In fact, television is worse than addiction to drugs, alcohol and cigarettes because over a billion or more people are addicted to it worldwide and few are unable to break their abuse.

So what does any of this have to do with asthma?

For decades the rate of asthma has been increasing in industrialized nations around the world, for both children and adults. There have been a lot of theories regarding this phenomenon, but no hard answers.

Air pollution is not the primary reason for the asthma increase. We know this because the asthma rate is increasing in cities where the level of pollution has actually decreased.

Indoor air pollution is a real possibility, as the number of hazardous home products has increased along with the population. Given the number of fragrance products, cleaning solvents, polishes, pesticides, personal care products, and volatile organic compounds that have entered our indoor air space over the decades, the culprit may indeed be in this realm.

Another possibility is that television acts as a catalyst in the presence of indoor pollutants, or it that it acts alone, independent of them. This is because of its role as another stressor. Below, I present possible ways in which television viewing can cause stress, leading to asthmatic symptoms in an otherwise relatively asymptomatic asthmatic person.

Advertising

Out of the 1,456 hours of TV watched per year, per person, approximately half that time is comprised of various breaks in the programming, most of which are related to advertising in one form or another. We watch someone yell at us with the volume increased, point their finger, cajole, promise, offer, entice, bribe, laugh, try to appear foolish, scare, intimidate, demonstrate, and otherwise strive to sell us their product or service. How many exercise machines can we buy? Who has the money? Where do we store them all? The same holds true for cookware.

It doesn't take a scientist to figure out that this leads to stress. We wouldn't permit those yelling persons to walk in our front door, but we watch them hour after hour on a vivid multicolored screen. Why do we do this? Let the psychologists answer that.

It is my opinion that spending money on the products that we want, but don't need, forces us into economic stress. I believe we are in debt as a nation because we are in debt as individuals. In a sense it's not our fault. We are being sold something we don't need.

Blurring the line between fantasy and reality

The news inflates the smallest issue into a national event. We are enticed to follow the sponsored coverage and to come right back after the commercial break. In the end, the program provides a format upon which even our dreams are based.

Unlike the exclusive use of radio, television has created a

generation of adults and children who lack imagination., The reason for this is that television presents the hype—a stressful exaggeration of events—in a manner that hooks and controls the viewer, conditioning us to expect exaggeration as demonstrated in car chase scenes, pyrotechnics (fires), and explosions. Thus, I believe, we either become apathetic to events in real life, or overreact. If we can't fathom the difference, then we are unquestionably victims of our times. Low voter turnout is only one example of our apathy, which is the measure of our apathy toward repeatedly bad judgment calls by political leaders who were voted in on their claims of trust.

Reducing creativity

Images fill our mind, as Jerry Mander so eloquently stated in his book *Four Arguments for the Elimination of Television*.[6] Jerry Mander had it right, but needed to go a step or two further.

His argument is valid in that the images are not those that result from creative thinking or original thought initiated by the viewer. They are somebody else's images. Depending on them instead of generating our own images makes us lethargic and less creative.

Some suggest that a world war is necessary to bring us out of our lethargy. I suggest that it only takes more and better writers and speakers. Yet these people, as well as classical composers and great painters, theoretically cannot be born anew in the era of the television. Perhaps, just as necessity is the mother of invention, so boredom can be the mother of creativity. While television purports to take away our boredom, it does just the opposite.

With great sadness I submit that television will not bow out with a curtsey, leaving our dignity or self-esteem intact, and exit the stage.

Therefore, the task that befalls us, as readers and as listeners, is to become as great as we can be, even in its midst.

Sleep deprivation

TV is not relaxing. It is just the opposite. If it were relaxing, we would be able to sleep well after watching hours of it each evening before bed. Poor sleep patterns mean more stress.

Violence and conflict

Watching violence and action leads to violent and active thoughts and behavior. This has been well researched and documented for decades.

By the time today's American is eighteen years old he will have viewed two hundred thousand acts of violence on TV. One can only imagine a perfect world where this many acts of kindness are performed instead.

Television is full of conflicts and overstimulation. Neither children nor adults are able to release the physical stress that they feel due to this overstimulation. Conflict resolution by this medium is miniscule compared with the stress it induces.

Indirect effects

a) An immune system that operates on a diet of TV dinners and fast food is not in a position to react well to allergens, b) The nervous system requires exercise, c) There is no minimum daily requirement for artificial lighting to enter our eyes.

For hours each day the television viewers don't see sunlight and don't read a book. Our next generation of leaders may not be able to read or write. Certainly, today's students can't. It is now a well-accepted fact that the art of handwriting is disappearing. These flaws increase the stress load for those job seekers who lack fundamental skills of mathematics and linguistics, the two skills most closely correlated with success in life.

The use of computers is not a stressor, per se. In my opinion, the use of computers is a great aid to those inventive persons who wish to further their knowledge. This knowledge is more available now than it ever was, thanks to the Internet. Research and availability of information become easier to obtain and the use of the computer can only help the educational and inventive process for those who do not abuse it.

Keeping us indoors

It is estimated that 85 percent of asthma has an allergic component. Studies have shown us that indoor air is much more polluted than outdoor air. For the reason that we spend more than 90 percent of our time indoors, we surround ourselves with toxic products that have been sold to us through advertising on TV.[5]

(Please read chapter 4, "We Are Covered in Chemicals.")

A cruel synergism occurs, an enhancing effect that television inflicts upon the viewer whose immune system is already assaulted by household products that are respiratory irritants, chemically derived foods, improper nutrition, and lack of exercise, to name a few. The end result is a worldwide increase in asthma in industrialized nations, those same nations that modernize their product lines and sell televisions to the masses.

Beyond asthma

When it is not providing solace to those who truly need it, television sucks up energy, time, money, creativity, vitality, and family life.

In turn, it provides transient and shallow entertainment that is short-lived. It also provides an opportunity for obesity to take root and causes sleeplessness and unpleasant dreams. It facilitates bad study habits, which presage bad grades in school. It makes a significant contribution toward a violent society, and importantly, for our purposes, provides the stress factors that trigger worsening asthma conditions in developing countries.

It wastes life.

I also believe that television is responsible for the increase in the cancer rate for many of the same reasons. But that's another story.

As for myself, I am not going to quit television cold turkey. But these days, the mute button is at hand and some project is in my lap, even as I cut down on viewing time.

Chapter 4

Pollen and Mold Data

The information presented below is meant to be a general guideline for aeroallergens for various cities in the United States. These data were obtained from numerous sources, including publications from the American Academy of Allergy, Asthma and Immunology and from numerous scientific papers. No attempt was made to review all the scientific literature. Therefore, this table is intended to serve in the most general comparative sense.

[The National Allergy Bureau (NAB™) is the section of the American Academy of Allergy, Asthma and Immunology's (AAAAI) aeroallergen network that is responsible for reporting current pollen and mold spore levels to the public.[1] With 78 counting stations in the United States they obtain regular and reliable information on the levels of these allergens for public information and its website is open to the public's perusal.]

The numbers presented are rounded off for easy reading. These figures depend upon the number of monitors available to a given city, and they can vary greatly from one area of a city to another, and from one year to the next. Unfortunately, there are problems with these data. The good news is that each count is collected from an allergist or from a university. The bad news is that only one area from each city is sampled. One area may not be representative of the entire city, but at least it follows.

There is another problem. Unless your pollen and mold data can be verified as having originated from your particular city, chances are that they are supplied by a paid-for company that uses twenty year averages. This is tantamount to the weatherman saying that the average weather of the day over a twenty-year period is seventy-two degrees when you note that a freezing rain is prevailing. For the reason that it is the weather of the day that determines the aeroallergen level, the data may be generally right, but specifically wrong.

Only the highest pollen and mold counts are presented in terms of number of particles per cubic meter per day. Because of the complicated names of molds, abbreviations are presented in most cases.

Numerous types of pollens and molds were omitted for the sake of simplicity. Virtually all of the cities listed were chosen because the type of monitor used was the same. Other cities were omitted from the listing because the type of monitor was different and the information could not be compared with the cities listed below.

ABBREVIATIONS

Cladosporium	Clado
Alternaria	Alt
Helminthosporium	Helmin
Fusarium	Fus
Aspergillus	Asp
Penicillium	Pen

The amount represents the average number of spores or pollen grains per cubic meter of air per 24-hour period.

Pollen and Mold Data Collected Nationally

POLLEN	Month	Amount	MOLD	Month	Amount
Albuquerque, NM					
Juniper	May	500	Clado	Nov	22,000
Ash	Apr	2,500	Helmin	June	300
Austin, TX					
Juniper	Jan	2,700	Clado	May	12,000
Oak	Apr	2,500	Alt	Aug	8,600
Elm	Sept	3,000	Asp	Sept	3,200
Ragweed	Oct	2,500			
Billings, MT					
Poplar	Apr	350	Clado	June	1,500
Grass	June	200	Smuts	July	2,300
Sagebrush	Sept	100	Helmin	Aug	100
Boise, ID					
Sycamore	May	450			
Sagebrush	Oct	550	no information available		
Boulder, CO					
Poplar	May	2,800	Clado	Aug	12,000
Grasses	June	2,600			
Ragweed	Aug	2,500			
Brooklyn, NY					
Oak	May	3,100	Clado	Aug–Sept	46,000
Sycamore	May	2,000	Pullularia	July	1,700
Hackberry	May	900	Fus	Aug	1,600
			Mush. spores	Aug–Sept	7,000

POLLEN	Month	Amount	MOLD	Month	Amount

Burlington, VT

POLLEN	Month	Amount	MOLD	Month	Amount
Birch	May	2,400	Clado	Sept	500
Ragweed	Aug	350	Mush. spores	Sept	33,000

Cape Girardeau, MO

POLLEN	Month	Amount	MOLD	Month	Amount
Oak	Apr	14,000	Alt	Sept	13,000
Elm	Mar	6,100	Clado	May	5,000
Maple	Apr	2,200			
Ragweed	Sept	6,400			

Clayton, MO

POLLEN	Month	Amount	MOLD	Month	Amount
Ragweed	Aug	2,500	Clado	Aug	14,000
Grasses	June	900	Mush. spores	Aug	25,000

Colorado Springs, CO

POLLEN	Month	Amount	MOLD	Month	Amount
Elm	May	26,000			
Poplar	May	11,000	no information available		
Ragweed	Aug	9,500			
Grasses	Aug	2,300			

Daytona Beach, FL

POLLEN	Month	Amount	MOLD	Month	Amount
Juniper	Feb	80	no information available		
Oak	Apr	80			

Des Moines, IA

POLLEN	Month	Amount	MOLD	Month	Amount
Ragweed	Aug	9,800	Clado	Aug–Sept	27,000
Nettle	Aug	1,100	Rusts	Sept	1,100
Grasses	June	750			

El Paso, TX

POLLEN	Month	Amount	MOLD	Month	Amount
Mulberry	Mar	5,700	Rusts	Aug	1,100
Juniper	Mar	1,100	Alt	Aug	700

POLLEN	Month	Amount	MOLD	Month	Amount
			Fresno, CA		
Olive	May	400	Clado	Sept	6,400
Grasses	June	900	Smuts-rusts	June	6,000
			Kalamazoo, MI		
Elm	Mar	125			
Mulberry	May	25	no information available		
Ragweed	Aug	140			
			La Jolla, CA		
Oak	Mar	250	Clado	Sept	11,000
Grasses	Aug	225			
			Mason City, IA		
Maple	May	150	Clado	Aug–Oct	160,000
Ragweed	Aug	3,700	Smuts	Oct	4,600
Grass	June	1,100			
			Minneapolis, MN		
Oak	May	1,500	Clado	July–Aug	12,000
Juniper	Apr	1,500			
Oak	May	2,300			
Ragweed	Aug				
			Newark, NJ		
Birch	May	250			
Oak	May	250	no information available		
Ragweed	Sept	50			
			Portland, ME		
Birch	May	2,100	Mush. Spores	July	1,900
Oak	May	1,800			
Ragweed	Aug	61			

POLLEN	Month	Amount	MOLD	Month	Amount
Providence, RI					
Oak	May	26,000	Clado	Aug	11,000
Birch	May	10,000	Fus	Aug	1,500
Ragweed	Sept	4,200	Curvularia	July–Aug	1,100
Reno, NV					
Juniper	Mar	50			
Elm	Mar	50	no information available		
Sagebrush	Oct	40			
Sacramento, CA					
Mulberry	Mar	12,000	Clado	Apr	9,000
Birch	Mar	200	Alt	Mar–Apr	1,500
Alder	Jan	150			
Grass	Mar	1,500			
San Diego, CA					
Oak	Apr	100			
Mulberry	Apr	20	no information available		
Grasses	June	15			
San Francisco, CA					
Juniper	Mar	350	Clado	Nov	70
Chestnut	May	100	Alt	May	50
Grass	May	400			
Saratoga, FL					
Oak	Mar	2,300	Clado	Sept	7,600
Aust. pine	Oct	300	Helmin	July	800
Palm	June	100			
Grasses	May–Aug	600			
Spokane, WA					
Pine	June	4,600	Smuts	June	7,200
Grasses	June	600	Clado	Aug	1,600

POLLEN	Month	Amount	MOLD	Month	Amount
			Tucson, AZ		
Mulberry	Mar	250	Clado	Oct	150
Olive	Apr	100	Alt	Oct	50
Ragweed	Mar	25	Smuts	May	35
Grasses	Sept	25			
			Tulsa, OK		
Elm	Mar	2,500	Clado	Sept	12,000
Oak	Apr	2,100	Pen	June	800
Poplar	Apr	1,900	Mush. spores	May	3,200
Ragweed	Sept	11,000			
Grasses	Apr	1,500			
			Washington DC		
Hickory	May	750	Alt	July–Aug	300
Birch	May	650	Fus	Aug	300
Oak	May	300			
Grass	June	200			

Additional notes: Juniper also includes cypress and cedar. Pine is not listed for space considerations and because it is minimally allergenic. When two or more months are listed, this means that the counts are about the same for each of the months.

Chapter 5

What is Synergism?

Most people know that synergism means that one plus one is more than two. In fact, like everything in science, it is more complicated than what it appears to be. The medical literature is rife with examples of chemically induced synergism. The Combination drug therapy has been used for decades in the treatment of cancer.

We are cautioned not to drink alcoholic beverages when we take medication. One reason for this is that we might neutralize the effect of the antibiotic (this is called antagonism) or we might enhance its effect because alcohol will permit greater entry of the medication into the cells of our body. Neither is good because the dosages for medications are worked out by the pharmaceutical companies on persons who are not taking alcohol.

In a simple example, one antibiotic may kill certain bacteria at a certain rate because it affects the cell wall of the bacteria. Add another antibiotic whose mode of action is to affect the bacterial DNA to a limited extent and combine the two. When the cell wall is compromised by antibiotic number one, it permits antibiotic number two to enter the cell at a great rate. The result is an enhanced killing effect on the bacteria. This is called synergism.

Synergism is based not just on the two or more ingredients, but upon their relative concentrations.

This is important for our purposes because it means that exposure to some chemicals that are present in a particular fragrance alone plus exposure to certain pesticides may mean that one plus one may equal ten or may also equal one thousand-fold effect on us. Other possible combinations are present: Fragrances plus certain foods; some pesticides used in combination with other pesticides; chemicals present in cleaning agents such as petroleum distillates plus fragrances plus allergenic foods; or allergies in general, plus cleaning products, just to name a few examples. In the latter case, our exposure to a certain fragrance(s) may cause an enhanced sensitivity to those allergens or even contribute to our reactions to the chemical(s) in the fragrance. Thus, depression, sleeplessness, excitement, irritability, and mood swings may all become more frequent and may occur with more intensity when two or more chemicals enter the body.

To complicate matters, three or more factors may interact to provide a synergistic effect, which may be positive or negative in their end result. For our purposes, it is the negative effects that are part of our everyday environment.

Chapter 6

The Spread of Viruses and Bacteria

At the risk of presenting an overly simplistic picture of the spread of respiratory related viruses, I will provide a few basics that, hopefully, will prevent the reader the misfortune of becoming infected during the course of their daily lives.

Respiratory viruses are named that because they infect the mucous lining of the respiratory tract, not necessarily because they are spread through respiration. They have two primary modes of infection. Certainly, under crowded conditions such as in a school, airline, office and other areas where the density of people is high, sneezing and exhalation of droplets is undoubtedly the mode of virus spread. Unfortunately, we still have not been able to conclusively prove that the virus is spread in this manner because the setting up of experiments to do so is extremely difficult.

Secondly, the virus also causes mucous drainage. A very high concentration of viruses is present in the droplets that easily find their way to the face and hands. Thus, when an infected person touches a surface such as a refrigerator and microwave handle, doorknob, supermarket rail, and market cart handles, we can expect a large number of virus particles to be transferred in this manner. When that finger or hand goes into the nose or mouth, the germs are transferred. When we use a glass that an infected person drank from, we can also expect virus transmission in that manner. This is called hand-to-mouth transfer or transfer through fomites.

In schools, studies have found that nearly 22 million school days are lost each year to the common cold and that some viruses and bacteria can live from 20 minutes up to 2 hours on door knobs and tables (desks).

After years of study, careful experiments that are set up to measure sneeze droplets reveal one thing: it is almost impossible to measure how many virus particles are being sprayed over what distance and how many of them are actually capable of being infectious.

Face masks are not effective against the inhalation of viruses, despite newspaper and television pictures of persons wearing them to protect against cold and flu viruses. This is because the virus particle is so small that it can readily pass through the pores of a filter and if the pore size of a filter is small enough to filter out a virus, a person would not be able to breathe. In fact, many believe the use of a face mask is detrimental to a person's cure because of reinfection by the same virus that is present in the moisture that has been deposited in the mask.

Bacteria such as *E. (Escherichia) coli, Salmonella,* and *Staphylococcus* may be inhaled occasionally, but they will not cause any disease in this method of exposure. Plague, tuberculosis, and Legionnaires disease are examples of three well known bacterial diseases transmitted by the respiratory route, although not necessarily exclusively by this route.

When a sewage flood occurs in the home, all states require certain cleanup methods and most require testing of surfaces for coliform bacteria (*E. coli* forms, including intestinal bacteria such as *Salmonella* and *Enterococcus*). However, as AIHA notes,[8] there has never been a case of disease transmission through the respiratory route due to this problem. Once the area is dried the bacteria will only survive for a matter of days, even if disinfection does not occur, although there may be pockets of bacteria that may remain if areas of moisture are not removed. It is the hand-to-mouth transmission of disease-causing agents that is of concern here. The use of heat and disinfectants are the two primary methods of cleanup in a sewage backup.

Chapter 7
Looking through the Microscope

I never have any expectations as to what I might find when I view an air sample at 300-600 magnification.

Along with carbon exhaust particles from vehicles, the powder from the wings of pigeons and doves is almost universally present indoors and outdoors, The powder comes in variable sizes, along with up to fifty other types of particulates. It would be embarrassing for me to tell you how many years it took me to recognize the origin of these powder particles.

The sample may reveal a high number of airborne mold spores that were supposed to be removed because of high technology air filtration. Or, a squirrel cage that operates commercial air scrubbers might be off center to result in the generation of thousands of respirable aluminum fragments that enter the air, even though the filter has removed other particles.

There are ways to compute the number of virtually any type of particulate. Once I know the volume of air and the number of minutes that I used to collect that volume, it is a simple matter to multiply the number of a particular particle type that I count times the number of liters of air that were obtained.

The fun part comes in determining whether the particles belong or don't belong. Three thousand particles (per cubic meter of air) of corn starch in a master bedroom is evidence that somebody is using a lot of body talc. If the person(s) has an allergy to corn, this could be an important discovery.

Mold is a little more difficult because there are so many mold genera and species that a person needs to be familiar with them. Fortunately, there are only a half-dozen or so that are common indoor contaminants of structural materials. Their type and number needs to be matched up with what is outdoors or in other areas of the home to arrive at a conclusion. The types of molds that are identified are more important than their number.

A total environmental inspection is the most fun. In one case I found fifteen thousand microscopic rust particles in the master bath of an asthma patient who was complaining of frequent attacks. The air ducts were rusted and lined with fiberglass, as well. Fiberglass particles were counted in the air samples. (I also found that he was using an inordinate number of fragrance products. The recommendations were obvious—clean the air ducts, install a bathroom fan, and switch to non fragrance home and personal care products. The results of these recommendations are pending.

On another occasion, I found 34 mold spores near an air purification machine and over 17,000 ten feet away. Since then, I began using more samplers for each job to get a more accurate picture of air turbulence factors in the processes involved in air filtration.

Pollen identification is also very interesting. For one thing, certain mold spores sharply increase in number one-two days prior to a major pollen outbreak. For another, sometimes a high pollen count can be found inside a building because of open doors and windows, lots of yard work going on, pollen laden clothing that is worn inside, or pollinating trees located just next to a window, and other factors.

Many times I don't know what I'm looking at. Plant particles look alike, although I know they are giving me clues as to their origin. I do know that whenever there is a fire somewhere in the world, say Indonesia, or Central America, or a volcano erupts, I can pick up particles of ash in my laboratory in Southern Arizona after they have traveled the world on the jet stream.

Looking through the microscope, I calculate that we inhale tens of millions to hundreds of millions of this witches brew of particles each day and I wonder how so few among them can cause us such grief. Just a few ragweed or grass pollen grains, say from ten to a hundred, will do the trick. New discoveries are being reported all the time regarding the ingredients of this stew.

Chapter 8
Proper Hand-washing

There is no question that handwashing can significantly reduce the spread of viruses and bacteria, but what constitutes proper handwashing?

According to the Centers for Disease Control and Prevention the following steps should be followed:

1. Hands should be washed using soap and warm, running water

2. Hands should be rubbed vigorously during washing for at least 20 seconds with special attention paid to the backs of the hands, wrists, between the fingers and under the fingernails (and beneath rings)

3. Hands should be rinsed well while leaving the water running

4. With the water running, hand should be dried with a single-use towel

5. Turn off the water using a paper towel, protecting washed hands to prevent re-contamination

Hands should be washed after the following activities:

1. After touching bare human body parts other than clean hands and clean, exposed portions of arms,

2. After using the toilet

3. After coughing, sneezing, using a handkerchief or disposable tissue, using tobacco, eating or drinking

4. After handling soiled equipment or utensils

5. Before food preparation, and after food preparation, as often as necessary to remove soil and contamination and to prevent cross-contamination when changing tasks (especially when preparing salads, meats and poultry)

6. After switching between working with raw food and working with ready-to-eat food and after engaging in other activities that contaminate the hands

(Author's note: Avoid touching face or inserting fingers into your mouth or nose at all times, but especially after touching public door handles, shopping cart handles, supermarket railings, and other areas that are handled by the public at large.)

7. Hand sanitizers containing 60-90 percent ethyl or isopropanol may be used as an adjunct to not as a replacement for proper handwashing.

Author's note: Commonly used public objects include market basket and checkout handles and railings, restroom door handles and exercise club weights and machines. Regarding restrooms, management should be encouraged to place a waste receptacle near the door for discard of waste paper towels.

Endnotes

1. Siple, PA and Passel, CF. 1945. Measurements of dry atmospheric cooling in subfreezing temperatures. Proc Am Philos Sci. 89:177-99.

2. Franz, R. 1998. New Insights about Sensitive Skin. *Dermatology Nursing.* Dec.

3. Connor, S. 2000. Women are far more sensitive to pain than men. *Science News.* The Independent. Feb.

4. Griffiths, J.F. *Climate and the Environment.*Paul Elk Publ. (London)1976.

5. U.S. Department of Education. 2008. Parents' Reports of the School Readiness of Young Children from the National Household Education Survery's Program of 2007. *National Center for Education Statistics.* Aug.

6. Mander, J. 1977. *Four Arguments for the Elimination of Television. How we Turn Into our Images.* Perennial Publishers, New York. 216

7. Vivian, J. The Media of Mass Communication. Allyn and Bacon Publ. 1991.

8. Field Guide for the Determination of Biological Contaminants in Environmental Samples. A publication of the American Industrial Hygiene Association. 2nd ed. AIHA Fairfax, VA. 2005, p. 100.

Suggested Reading

Key to journal abbreviations

Acad	Academy
Allerg	Allergy
Amer	American
Ann	Annals
Arch	Archives
Chem	Chemical
Clin	Clinical
Contam	Contamination
Emer	Emergency
Engin	Engineering
Env	Environmental
Exp	Experimental
Expos	Exposure
Immunol	Immunology
Ind	Industry
Int	Internal
J	Journal
Med	Medicine
Occup	Occupational
Onc	Oncology
Persp	Perspectives
Proc	Proceedings
Resp	Respiratory
Rev	Review
Tox	Toxicology

Al-Doory, Y. and J.F. Domson. 1984. Mould Allergy and Climate Conditions, by Mark R. Sneller. *In: Mould Allergy*. Lea and Febiger, Philadelphia. 244-266.

Al-Saleh I. 1994. Pesticides: A Review Article. *J Env Path Tox Onc.* 13(3):151

Alawi M.A., F. Khalill and I. Sahali. 1994. Determination of Trihalomethanes Produced Through the Chlorination of Water as a Function of its Humic Acid Content. *Arch Env Contam Tox.* 26:381

Anderson, RC and JH Anderson. 1998. Acute Toxic Effects of Fragrance Products. *Arch Environ Health.* Mar-Apr;53(2):138-46

Aristatek. 2006. Hydrogen Cyanide Poisoning from Inhalation of Smoke Produced in Fires. *The First Responder Newsletter.* April

Arlian, L. et al. 1992. Prevalence of Dust Mites in the Homes of People with Asthma Living in Eight Different Geographic Areas of the United States. *J Allerg Clin Immunol.* 90(3):292.

Ashford, N. and C. Miller. 1991. *Chemical Exposures — Low Levels and High Stakes.* Van Norstrand Reinhold.

Babin, A., P. Peltz and M. Rossol. 1992. Risky Art Supplies: 13 Safe Substitutes. Adapted from "Art Materials: Recommendations for Children Under 12." *Center for Safety in the Arts.*

Bardana Jr. E. and A. Montanaro. 1991. Formaldehyde: An Analysis of its Respiratory, Cutaneous, and Immunologic Effects *Ann Allerg.* 66:441.

Bardana, Jr. E. and A. Montanaro. 1997. *Indoor Air Pollution and Health*. Marcel Decker, Inc.

Berthold-Bond, A. 1990. Clean and Green. Ceres Press.

Bollinger ME, et al. 1996. Cat Antigen in Homes with and Without Cats May Induce Allergic Symptoms. *J Allerg Clin Immunol*. 97(4):907.

Bower, J. 1997. Healthy House Building—A Design and Construction Guide. The Healthy House Institute, Bloomington, IN.

Bush, RK, M.D. and PA Eggleston, M.D. 2001. Guidelines for Control of Indoor Allergen Exposure. *J Allerg Clin Immunol*. 107(3):S403.

Camcioglu, Y., M.D. and H Cokugras, M.D. 2000. Local and Systematic Reactions During Immunotherapy with Adsorbed Extracts of House Dust Mite in Children. *Ann of Allergy, Asthma & Immunol*. Oct;85(4)317-21

Chang, D. M.D. et al. 1993. The Building Syndrome. I. Definition and Epidemiological Considerations. *J Asthma*. 30(4):285.

Chang, D. M.D. et al. 1994. The Sick Building Syndrome. II. Assessment and Regulation of Indoor Air Quality. *J Asthma*. 30(4):297.

Chang, D. M.D. et al. 1994. Building Components Contributors of the Sick Building Syndrome. *J Asthma*. 31(2)127.

Chapman, M.D. and R.A. Wood, M.D. 2001. The Role and Remediation of Animal Allergens in Allergic Diseases. *J Allerg Clin Immunol.* 107(3):S414.

Chen, BH et al. 1997. Air Pollution: The Changing Perception of Health Risks, editorial. *Indoor Built Environment.* 6:1.

Cone, J.E. and D. Shusterman. 1991. Health effect of indoor odorants. *Env. Health Perspec.* 95:53.

Dadd, D.L. 1990. *Non-Toxic, Natural, and Earthwise.* St. Martin's Press, NY.

DeFrance, T. 2006. A review: Health Symptoms Caused by Molds in a Courthouse., by Lee, T.G. Arch Environ Health July 2005 58:7 Symptoms Caused by Molds, *in* Our Toxic Times, Aug.

Department of Mechanical and Aerospace Engineering. 2004. Effectiveness of portable air cleaners for control of volatile organic compounds in indoor air. Syracuse University, NY. Publ. in *Our Toxic Times.* October. (See Chemical Injury Information Network or CIIN website at CIIN.com.

Eggleston, P.A. M.D. and R.K. Bush M.D. 2001. Environmental allergen avoidance: An overview. *J Allerg Clin Immunol.* 107(3):S403.

Emmons, CW, et al. 1977. Medical Mycology. Lea and Febiger, Phila. 3rd ed.

EPA. Formaldehyde.(50-00-0)

EPA. 1987. Inert Ingredients in Pesticide Products. *Policy State-ment.* EPA/ 0PP-36140;FRL-3190-1

EPA. *Questions and Answers on Lawn Pesticides.* http://pmep.cce.cornell.edu/issues/lawnissues.html

EPA. 1989. *Inert Ingredients in Pesticide Products; Policy Statement; Revision and Modification of Lists.* EPA/0PP-36140;FRL-3190-1

EPA. 1995. *List of Pesticide Product Inert Ingredients.*

Essential Ozone. Alpine Industries. 9199 Central Avenue NE., Minn., Minn.

Ewers, L. et al. 1994. Clean up of lead in household carpet and floor dust. *Amer Ind Hyg Assoc J.* 55:650.

Fagin, D., M. Lavelle, and the Center for Public Integrity. 1996. Toxic Deception—How the Chemical Industry Manipulates Science, Bends the Law, and Endangers your Health. *Inerts.* Carol Publishing Group, Secaucus

Felix K. et al. 1996. Allergens of Horse Dander: Comparison among breeds and Individual Animals by Immunoblotting. *J Allerg Clin Immunol.* 98(1):169.

Flegal, AR and DR Smith. 1995. Measurement of Environmental Lead. *Rev Env Contam Tox.* Springer. 6-11.

Frey, A. 1996. Enhancing Contaminant Control to Mitigate Aeroallergens. *Ann Allergy Asthma Immunol.* 77:460.

Geno, PW et al. 1996. Handwipe Sampling and Analysis Procedure for the Measurement of Dermal Contact with Pesticides. *Arch Environ Contam Tox*. 30:132.

Gerbner, G. and L. Gross. 1976. The Scary World of TV's Heavy Viewer. *Psychology Today*. April

Godish, T. 1989. Indoor Air Pollution Control. Lewish Publ. Chelsea, MI.

Gotz, IL. 1975. On Children and Television. *Elementary School Journal*. April, 415-418

Green, J. 2001. *Magic Brands: 1185 Brand-New Uses for Brand Name Products*. Rodale Inc.

Harte, J. et al. 1991. *Toxics A to Z. A Guide to Everyday Pollution Hazards*. Univ. of California Press.

Hasenauer R.F. et al. 1996. Formaldehyde Exposure Enhances Inhalative Allergic Sensitization in the Guinea Pig. *J. Allerg*. 51:94.

Jelks, M. M.D. 1987. *Allergy Plants That Cause Sneezing and Wheezing*. World-Wide Printing PO Box 24339, Tampa FL 33623 ISBN: 0-911977-04-X

Jones, A.P. 2000. Asthma and the home environment. Review Article. *J Asthma*. 37(2):103.

Katsarou A, M.D., et al. 1999. Contact reactions to fragrances. *Ann Allerg Asthma Immun*. 82:449.

Kelly, F. et al. 1995. The free radical basis of air pollution: Focus on ozone. *Resp Med.* 89:647

Krishna, M.T. et al. 1995. Ozone, airways and allergic airways disease. *Clin Exp Allerg.* 25:1150.

Lansky, V. 1995. Baking Soda. Over 500 Fabulous Fun and Frugal Uses You've Probably Never Thought Of. Book Peddlers.

Lemier, C. et al. 1996. Occupational asthma caused by aromatic herbs. *Allerg.* 51:647.

Lewis, R.G., R.C. Fortmann and D.E. Camann. 1994. Evaluation of methods for monitoring the potential exposure of small children to pesticides in the residential enviornment. *Arch Environ Contam Tox.* 26:37

Lewis, RD and PN Breysse. 2000. Carpet Properties that Affect the Retention of Cat Allergen. *Ann Allergy, Asthma & Immun.* Jan;84(1)31-36

Linden, S. 1996. A Review of: Sensitivity to Electricity-A New Environmental Epidemic. *Allergy.* 51:519-524.

Lindgren, S., M.D. et al. 1988. Breed-spectific Dog-Dandruff Allergens. *J Allerg Clin Immunol.* 82(2):196.

Lioy, PJ and E. Pellizzari 1995. Conceptual Framework for Designing a National Survey of Human Exposure. *J Exp Analysis Env Epid.* 5(3):425

Lioy, P. et al. 1998. The Effectiveness of a Home Cleaning Intervention Strategy in Reducing Potential Dust and Lead Exposures. *J Expos Anal Env Epid.* 8(1):17.

Logan, K. 1997. *Clean House, Clean Planet.* Pocket Books.

Lewis R.D. and P.N. Breysse. 2000. Carpet Properties that Affect the Retention of Cat Allergen. *Ann Allerg Asthma Immunol.* 84:31

Lion, D. *Creating a Safe Fragrance-Free Environment That's Healthy for All of Us.* www.bpf.org/html/whats_now/MCSResources.

Lu P. 1992. A Health Hazard Assessment in School Arts and Crafts. *J Env Path Tox Onc.* 11:12.

Marshall PS and EA Colon, M.D. 1993. Effects of Allergy Season on Mood and Cognitive Function. *Ann Allerg.* 71:251.

Maryland Department of Agriculture, Pesticide Regulation Section. 2001. *MDA Pesticide Information Sheet.* Reducing off Target Movement of Pesticides Indoors. MDA 145 No. 18

McCants M., et al. 2000. The Effects of Fragrances on Respiratory Reactions of Asthmatics. *Amer Acad of Allerg, Asthma Immunol.* 56th Annual Meeting, Abstract No. 371.

Molfino, N. et al. 1991. Effect of Low Concentrations of Ozone on Inhaled Allergen Responses in Asthmatic Subjects. *Lancet* 1991, 338.

National Air Duct Cleaners Association. 1992-01. *Guideline to NADCA Standard*, 1518 K Street, N.W., Suite 503, Wash. D.C. 20005.

National Cancer Institute. 2004. *Radon and Cancer: Questions and Answers. Fact Sheet.* www.cancer.gov/cancertopics/fact-sheet/risk/radon

Ormstad, H. et al. 1998. Airborne House Dust Particles and Diesel Exhaust Particles as Allergen Carriers. *Clin Exp Allerg.* 28:702.

Ort, W.R. and J.W. Roberts. 1998. Everyday Exposure to Toxic Pollutants. *Scientific Amer.* (Feb):86.

Palmer. 1976. *Body Weather: How Natural and Man-Made Climates Affect You and Your Health.* Stackpole Books, Harriburg, PA.

Peden, DB, M.D. et al. 1997. Prolonged Acute Exposure to 0.16 ppm Ozone Induces Eosinophilic Airway Inflammation in Asthmatic Subjects with Allergies. *J Allerg Clin Immunol* 100(6):802.

Peterson B. and A. Saxon. 1996. Global Increases in Allergic Respiratory Disease: The Possible Role of Diesel Exhaust Particles. *Ann. Allerg. Asth. Immunol.* 77:263.

Platts-Mills T. et al. 1997. Indoor Allergens and Asthma: Report of the Third International Workshop. *J Allerg Clin Immunol.* 100(6):S2

Platt-Mills T., M.D. and M. Chapman M.D. 1987. Dust mites:

Immunology, Allergic Disease, and Environmental Control. *J Allerg Clin Immunol.* 80(6):755.

Price, S. 1993. *The Aromatherapy Workbook.* Hammersmith, London, Thorsons

Radetsky, P. 1997. *Allergic to the Twentieth Century.* Little, Brown and Co.

Rapp, DJ M.D. 1996. Is This Your Child's World? How you Can Fix the Schools and Homes that are making your Children Sick. Bantam Books.

Rinzler, CA. 1980. *The Consumer's Brand-Name Guide to Household Products.* Lippincott and Crowell.

Roberts JW et al. 1992. Human Exposure to Pollutants in the Floor Dust of Homes and Offices. *J Expos Anal Environ Epid Suppl.* 2:127.

Roberts JW et al. 1993. Chemical Contaminants in House dust: Occurrences and Sources. *Indoor Air.* Proceedings of the 6th International Conference on Air Quality and Climate Vol. 2:27. Helsinki University of Technology. Espoo, Finland.

Roberts, JW, et al. 1995. Measurement of Deep Dust and Lead in Old Carpets. Measurement of Toxic and Related Pollutants. *Proc Air and Waste Management Assn,* San Antonio, TX.

Roberts JW and P. Dickey. 1995. Exposure of Children to Pollutants in House Dust and Indoor Air. *Rev Env Contam Tox.* 143:59.

Ronborg, SM, M.D. et al. 1999. Effect of Two Different Types of Vacuum Cleaners on Airborne Fel d 1 Levels. *Ann Allerg Asthma Immunol* 82:307.

Rosen, SM 1979. *Weathering: How the Atmosphere Conditions your Body, your Mind—and your Health*. Evans and Company, NY.

Rousseau, D., et al. 1988. *Your Home, Your Health, and Well-Being*. Hartley and Marks.

Scarfi, A. 2007. Anthony's Answers to Air Filtration. *Ecologic News*. Human Ecology Action league (HEAL). 24:4

Schlosser, E. 2001. *Fast Food Nation: The Dark Side of the All American Meal*. Houghton Mifflin.

Seargeant, SE 1997. *Allergy Free Living*. Serargent Publ. Co., Visalia, CA.

Shim, C, M.D. and M.H. Williams, Jr., M.D, 1986. Effect of Odors in Asthma. *Amer J Med*. 80:18.

Simmon, F., M.D. 1996. Learning Impairment and Allergic Rhinitis. *Allerg Asthma Proc*. 17:4.

Smedley, J. 1996. Is Formaldehyde an Important Cause of Allergic Respiratory Disease? Editorial. *Clin Exp Allerg* 26:247

Sneller, M.R., et al. 1977. Comparative study of Trichothecin, Amphotericin B and 5-Fluorocytosine against *Cryptococcus neoformans* in vitro and in vivo. *Antimicrob. Ag. Chemother.* 12:390

Sneller, M.R., et al. 1979. Incidence of Fungal Spores in an Agricultural Community. III. Associations with Local Crops. *Ann. Allergy.* 43:352,

Sneller, M.R.,et al. 1993. Pollen Changes During Five Decades of Urbanization in Tucson, Arizona. *Ann. Allergy* 71:519

Sorenson, W.G., et al. 1975. Qualitative and Quantitative Assay of Trichothecin: a Mycotoxin Produced by *Trichothecium roseum. Appl Microbiol* 29:653

Stellman, JM, M.D. and SM Daun, M.D. 1990. *Work is Dangerous to Your Health.* Vintage Books.

The Alert: *Allergy to Latex Education and Resource Team, Inc.* P.O. Box 23722, Milwaukee, WI 53223-0722.

The Human Ecology Action League, Inc. (HEAL). 1996. Multiple Chemical Sensitivity and the Americans with *Disabilities Act. A Guide to Accessibility.* Atlanta, GA, Ph. 404-248-1898.

Tubiolo VC, and GN Beall. 1997. Clin Dog Allergy: Understanding our 'Best Friend'? *Exp Allerg.* 27:354.

Turner, W. et al. 1995. Ventilation. *Occup Med.* 10(1):41.

Turner, S. et al. 1996. *Sources and Factors Affecting Indoor Emissions from Engineered Wood Products: Summary and Evaluation of Current Literature.* June EPA/600/SR-96/067.

Tuthill, R. 1996. Hair Lead Levels Related to Children's

Classroom Attention-Deficit Dehavior. Arch Env Health 51(3):214.

Wallace LA. 1991. Comparison of Risks from Outdoor and Indoor Exposure to Toxic Chemicals. *Environ Health Persp.* 95:7.

Wallace, LA. 1995. Human Exposure to Environmental Pollutants: A Decade of Experience. U.S. EPA. *Clin Exp Allerg.* 25:4.

Weiller JM, et al. Asthma in United States Olympic Athletes who Participated in the 1996 Summer Games. *J Allerg Clin immunol.* 102:722.

Whitmore, RW., et al. 1994. Non-Occupational Exposures to Pesticides for Residents of Two U.S. Cities. *Arch Env Contam Tox* 26:47.

Wilson, JW, MD and OR Plunkett, *The Fungous Diseases of Man.* 1967. University of California Press, Berkeley.

Winkless N. and I. Browning. 1975. *Climate and the Affairs of Men.* Harper and Row, NY.

Winter, RMS. 1994. *A Consumer's Dictionary of Cosmetic Ingredients.* Three Rivers Press.

Videos

1. Rapp, D.J., M.D., *Environmentally Sick Schools, Students and Teachers at Risk.* Practical Allergy Research Foundation. (Call 1-800-787-8780) 90 minutes

2. Xenejenex Health Care Communications Companies. *Coping with Allergies: Your Guide to Quick Relief From Sneezing, Coughing and Congestion.* Xenegenex Health Videos. Call 1-800-228-2495.

Glossary

AC: air conditioner (air conditioning)

Acetylcholine: a neurotransmitter in the peripheral nervous system and the central nervous system

Acid reflux: a condition in which the contents of the stomach (acid) and even bile from the small intestine back up into the esophagus to cause burning. There are numerous causes of this disorder including overeating or eating spicy foods

Acrylate copolymer: also known as acrylamide/sodium acrylate copolymer—used in moisturizers and other products; may be carcinogenic, if used at a high concentration

Activated charcoal: charcoal made from a variety of sources that have the ability to absorb contaminants from the air or the water within a network of charged microscopic lattices within the particle; used in air purifiers, fish tanks, layering on potting soil and a myriad of other uses; it is much more effective when crushed

Air fresheners: masking agents that contain essential oils and aromatic chemicals and which may deaden the sense of smell

Allergen: a particle that can cause an allergic reaction

Allergic: a person who has an allergy to a particle such as pollen or dust

Allergy: a disease of the immune system that is characterized by sneezing, itching of eyes, mucous drainage in the throat and sinus headaches; commonly caused by particles or foods

Angina: A disease marked by spasmodic attacks of intense suffocative pain

Anneal: to strengthen and toughen through the use of heat

Antibiotics: chemicals produced by mold(s) and bacteria that can inhibit the growth of other microorganisms, but have few harmful effects on the human (penicillin is one of several exceptions in which severe allergic reactions can occur)

Anticholinergics: chemical agents that are used to counteract the effect of the neurotransmitter acetylcholine in the peripheral and central nervous systems. Use for the treatment of asthma and chronic bronchitis and other disorders

Anther: the part of a flower that produces pollen

Antihistamine: drugs used to block the effects of histamine, and thus reduce the severity of allergic and asthmatic attacks

Asphyxiant: asphyxiant gases are non toxic or minimally toxic and displace oxygen to cause suffocation in confined spaces, e.g.,carbon dioxide

Asthma: a disease that is characterized by swelling and constriction of the airways, making breathing difficult

Asthmagenic: capable of causing symptoms of asthma

Asthmatic: a person who has asthma

ASHRAE: American Society of Heating, Refrigeration and Air Conditioning Engineers

Arteriolsclerosis: hardening of the or loss of elasticity of arteries

Atherosclerosis: a buildup of plaque within the arteries, usually comprised of cholesterol

Bacteria: a wide variety of microorganisms, of which many are beneficial and others are harmful; include staphylococcus (staph) and streptococcus (strep), and most of the well known diseases of man

Baking soda: (also known as sodium bicarbonate) is a naturally occurring white crystalline powder that is readily available and inexpensive; it has hundreds of uses, especially for odor removal in refrigerators, shoes, and for washing walls and cabinets to remove surface grime and VOCs; also used in the clothes washing machine, it is a natural buffer, neutralizing odors in the mouth and is used as a toothpaste, stain, and plaque remover.

Benign: generally without complications and with a good prognosis

Bergamot: an essential oil derived from a citrus fruit, used for treatment of acne, depression and stress as a few of many possible uses; asthmagenic

Beta adrenergic agonists: Beta 1 agonists are used as cardiac stimulants, Beta 2 agonists are used to treat asthma and COPD

Boric acid: an inexpensive naturally occurring white powder that readily dissolves in water; used as an antiseptic, insecticide and flame retardant; effective on sunburns and windburns, minor cuts, insect bites and effective against cockroaches, ants, fleas and silverfish

Bronchodilators: short or long acting medications that open up the bronchial tubes in asthma treatment and also act to clear mucus from the lungs

Carbonless copy paper: made with micro-encapsulated color formers on the back and color formers on the front of the paper sheets

Cajeput: an essential oil which is used for sore throat, rheumatism and asthma; contains limene and pinene; both classed as terpenes and can be asthmagenic when burned

Cat antigen: small molecular weight proteins associated with cat saliva and sebaceous glands; highly antigenic and long lasting in the home (or school); difficult to remove from the indoor environment; almost universally present

Chloramine: used as ammonium chloride in municipal water systems as a more stable replacement for chlorine; will react with organic tissue to create carbon tetrachloride and chloroform (both are considered to be toxic and carcinogens by the EPA; asthmagenic chloramine gas is formed with ammonia is mixed with chlorine containing cleaning agents.

Chloroform: once a widely used anesthetic, it is now considered a carcinogenic gas produced by the action of chlorine and ammonia in combination of organic tissue

CIIN: Chemical Injury Information Network

Circadian rhythm: daily cycles of growth exhibited by all life forms including biological, physiological and behavioral patterns; triggered by external factors such as sunlight

Corticosteroids: or steroids are powerful chemicals that resemble cortisol produced by the adrenal cortex; used in the treatment of arthritis and other inflammatory diseases, but have many adverse side effects which include the interference of white blood cell action, thus increasing the susceptibility to disease

Cromolyn: a synthetic chemical that prevents the release of histamine and other chemicals from mast cells

CRI: Carpet and Rug Institute

CS: chemical sensitivity

Cutaneous: relating to the skin

Cypress: an essential oil which is used for treatment of oily skin, rheumatism and asthma; contains pinene; can be asthmagenic when burned

Dander: skin cells

Decane: a ten carbon flammable liquid found in gasoline and produced as a byproduct of growth by some fungi

Dehumidifier: An electrical device that removes moisture from the air such as in basements and flooded homes

Diphasic fungi: cause histoplasmosis (histo), blastomycosis (blasto), and coccidioidomycosis (cocci) or San Joaquin Valley Fever); they have one form of spores in the ground and change to another form of spores in the human body

Dissemination: to spread from a central source, as in the dissemination of a fungus or other microbial agent from the lungs to other parts of the body

EC: evaporative cooler; a cooling device used in numerous states that blows air over water saturated aspen or cellulose fibers to bring cool air indoors

Eczema: various forms of dryness and rashes of the surface of the skin or epidermis; a form of dermatitis

Egress: to leave an area

Emulsifiers: additives used to keep substances together in solution that might normally separate, such as water and oil

Eosinophil: a type of white blood cell; can increase in number during an allergic reaction

Essential oils: Between 100 and 400 naturally occurring oils and their derivatives (depending on how they are classified) including spearmint, coffee, dill, lime, eucalyptus, vanilla and tea tree; used for aromatherapy as in burning through use of incense, chewing (gum or leaves), eating and drinking, or by direct application to the skin; each has medicinal properties ascribed to it; many are asthmagenic

Eucalyptus: an essential oil which is used for treatment of flu and coughing; contains pinene and limonene; can be asthmagenic when burned or smelled

Frankincense: an essential oil which is used for treatment of stretch marks, coughing, bronchitis, asthma; contains limonene and pinene; can be asthmagenic when burned or smelled

Hemoglobin: the iron containing protein of the blood that carries oxygen from the lungs to the rest of the body in humans and other; has other functions in other vertebrates

Hotspot: an area of microbial or VOC concern such as the refrigerator, a moldy wall, or the master bathroom

Humidifier: a device that produces cold or hot water mist to add moisture to the air

Humidistat: a sensor associated with a humidifier that senses the amount of humidity in the air and controls the operation of the humidifier; frequently inaccurate, since it only senses the humidity near the humidifier and not at more distant points

Formaldehyde: produced by virtually all life forms as a product of growth; a small molecule that is created synthetically and has hundreds of applications; outgases readily; a known eye and respiratory irritant at extremely low concentrations (0.01 – 1.0 ppm) outgases most when products are new and temperature and humidity are elevated; outgases slowly (as long as years) when little fresh air is present such as within cupboards and where temperatures are cooler and moisture is reduced

FTC: Federal Trade Commission

Fumes: vapors (gases) and particles emitted from the burning of various substances such as auto exhaust and fires

Fungi: a large group of microorganisms that include molds, mushrooms, plant pathogens such as smuts, which attack grains, and diphasic fungi

Ghosting: the effect of carbon soot particles produced by candle burning—the particles follow magnetic lines of force in a home to create unusual shapes on the walls and ceilings, in addition to causing a darkening of the walls

Half-life: The amount of time it takes one half of a given amount of substance to decay

HEAL: Human Ecology Action League

HEPA: High efficiency particulate air—a filter that can remove 99.97 percent of particles at a level of 0.3 microns (smaller than most bacteria), but not small enough to filter out viruses which can be ten times smaller than this.

Heredity: genetic factors that are inherited by ones parents, grandparents, and previous generations; carried in the DNA

Holding time: the time in which air or water is held in contact with decontaminants such as activated charcoal or ultraviolet light; the longer the holding time, the greater the efficiency of the agent

HVAC: Heating, ventilation and air conditioning

Hypersensitivity pneumonitis: an allergic reaction; an inflammation of the air sacs (alveoli) within the lungs caused by hypersensitivity to inhaled organic dusts such as bacteria, molds, fungi and even inorganic material; sufferers are frequently exposed through their professions or their hobbies; symptoms include fever and body ache, and difficulty in breathing

Hyposensitization: the use of injections to decrease the sensitivity to allergens; tailored to the individual; small doses are introduced to result in reduction in reactions

Hyssop: an essential oil used for the treatment of bruises, coughing, sore throat and asthma; contains limonene; asthmagenic

Idiopathic: any disease of unknown origin

IgE: immunoglobulin E or allergic antibody; present in mast

cells and basophils that serves to prime them to release histamine and other mediators upon exposure to allergens

IICRC: Institute of Inspection Cleaning and Restoration Certi-
fication

Inerts: may constitute over 99 percent of the ingredients in various products such as pesticides; used to extend the shelf life
of the product, enhance its stability in the presence of sunlight,
or to give the active ingredient more potency; "inert" does not
mean harmless, as believed by the public at large; since 1997
the EPA had encouraged companies to use the term "other ingredients" instead

Infiltrometer: a computerized device for determining where
air leakages occur within a home and the extent of the leakages

Ingress: to enter, the act of entering

Insidious: a gradual and cumulative effect as in development
of a disease state until symptoms are noted

Kapok: silky fibers from the seeds of a tropical tree used for
padding in pillows, mattresses, sleeping bags, and other products

Lavender: an essential oil which is used for headaches, various
skin disorders, asthma, and as an insect repellent; asthmagenic

Lime: an essential oil which is used for varicose veins, acne,

and asthma; contains limonene and pinene; can be asthmagenic when burned or smelled

Limonene: d-limonene is an oil present in the rind of citrus
fruit, especially oranges, lemons and limes; touted to reduce
the formation of cancer-causing cells; is used as a solvent and
cleaner; may have anti-mosquito properties; may be a respiratory irritant to some asthmatics and MCS patients

Mast cells: tissues cells rich in histamine and heparin (antico-
agulant); important in the allergic response and in wound healing

MCS: Multiple chemical sensitivity

Meninges three membranes that surround the brain and spinal cord and which contain cerebral spinal fluid

Mercaptan: a chemical in which the oxygen in an alcohol is replaced by a sulfur to produce a disagreeable odor; commonly
used as an odorant in natural gas lines to detect the presence
of leakages

Methylxanthines: a class of naturally occurring chemicals that
contain caffeine (e.g., coffee, cocoa, chocolate) and promote
smooth muscle relaxation and helps dilate restricted airways;

Mimeograph: a mechanical duplicator that produces copies by
pressing ink through a stencil

Mites: extremely tiny insects that are related to spiders and
commonly found in dust and which shed tremendous quanti-

ties of fecal pellets that are highly allergenic; present in more humid climates and found in soft furnishings including bedding

Mold(s): a large group of microorganisms that are present in soil and can contaminate water damaged buildings, vegetation in general, crops and produce; their spores are often allergenic, but less so than pollen

MSDS: Material Safety Data Sheet

Mycotoxin: toxic chemicals produced by many common fungi when growing on plants (ergot), and other foodstuffs such as grains and grasses that cause various symptoms of poisoning when ingested by humans and animals; not yet proved to be problematic when spores are inhaled

Myrrh: an essential oil which is used for athlete's foot, halitosis, asthma, and hemorrhoids; contains limonene; can be asthmagenic when burned or smelled

NAS: National Academy of Sciences

NCEHS: National Center for Environmental Health Strategies

Opacity: a measurement of the degree to which light is blocked

Oriented strand board: three layers of irregular shaped flakes of wood that range in size from one to six inches and bonded together with urea or phenol-formaldehyde to create plywood sheets, subflooring, underlayment for roofs, framing of homes, and numerous household products; more resistant to water and mold growth than pressed wood and made from rapidly growing trees harvested in special growth areas; touted as being environmentally friendly

OSB: Oriented strand board

Out-gas or outgas: the emission of gas from a product, such as formaldehyde outgassing from textile products

Ozonation: the use of ozone to kill microbes in water; its use as an antimicrobial in occupied buildings is debated; hazardous to breathe in higher concentrations

ppb: parts per billion (one part in a billion of air or water)

ppm: parts per million (one part in a million of air or water)

Paraffin: a wax made from vegetable or synthetic oils; used in candles and as a preservative; used to shine to fruits, vegetables, and chocolate

Passive electrostatic air filter: attains a negative charge when air passes through it and attracts positively charged dust particles; relatively inefficient

Perchloroethylene: a non-flammable toxic degreasing chemical used in the commercial dry cleaning of clothes; contaminates the air space within a closet since it evaporates from clothing upon exposure to air

Petroleum distillates: colorless solvents obtained from the distillation of petroleum used in a wide variety of household products from polishes to grease cutters; when used indoors, they can produce a high level of VOCs

Phenol-formaldehyde: also known as Bakelite; a resin used in a manner similar to urea-formaldehyde it is used in the manufacture of OSB for construction and outgases less than does UF

Picocuries: a measure of radiation

Pinene: present in the oil of pine trees and other conifers and has the pine scent; it is made from terpentine; can be used to make camphor and is a disinfectant and used as a fragrance; as a VOC, it is a respiratory irritant to perhaps millions of persons

Pressed wood: a product made from wood veneers, small particles and fibers bonded with urea formaldehyde; the finished product is used in the creation of numerous products for the home including furniture, vanities, and shelving; easily damaged by water (it swells and chips) and readily supports active mold growth

Psychosomatic: a concern for bodily symptoms caused by mental or emotional disturbance

R value: a measure of the resistance of an insulating or building material to heat flow; the higher the R value, the greater the resistance

Solvent: a liquid in which other liquids or solids are dissolved

Sonication: the use of high frequency sound to disrupt microbial cells and cause fragmentation of particles when they are present in liquids; used in some home humidifiers as an antimicrobial agent that may compound the problem by permitting still smaller particles to enter the air

Spearmint: an essential oil which is used for headache, fatigue and asthma; contains limonene and pinene; can be asthmagenic when burned or smelled

Spruce: an essential oil which is used for coughing, depression and asthma; contains limonene and pinene; can be asthmagenic when burned or smelled

Styrene: A derivative of benzene used in the manufacture of insulating materials (Styrofoam), carpet backing, plastic, rubber, and other products.

Surfactants: lower the surface tension of liquids, e.g., to permit better penetration of a cleaning agent into dirty articles of clothing

Swamp cooler: evaporative cooler

Synergy: the process whereby two or more chemicals or other agents have a multiplier rather than an additive effect

Thunderstorm asthma: An episode of asthma that occurs during and shortly after a thunderstorm.

Trisodium phosphate: an inexpensive powder readily available in hardware stores that is commonly used as a cleaning agent, stain remover and degreaser; used for cleaning sidings, walls prior to painting, and for removal of oil stains from concrete

TSP: trisodium phosphate

UF: Urea-formaldehyde

Urea formaldehyde: a thermosetting resin or plastic used in finishes and adhesives and used in the manufacture of pressed wood products; created when formaldehyde and urea are combined and heated in the presence of a catalyst; becomes easily damaged when wet and readily supports active mold growth

Vapors: gases emitted from various products

Vasomotor rhinitis: a non allergic reaction of the nose to viruses, bacteria, or irritants—characterized by drainage and sneezing and may occur seasonally or perennially

Virus: a non-living microbe that must use living cells to reproduce; found to infect virtually every type of life including bacteria, algae, fungi, plants, mammals, birds, fish, and insects

VOC: volatile organic compounds; liquids or solids that give off odorous gases such as glues, solvents, paints, nail polish remover, formaldehyde, ammonia, petroleum distillates

White spirit: known as Stoddard solvent; a degreaser and a solvent used in paint thinners, lacquers, varnishes, asphalt and wood preservatives

Yeasts: numerous species of single-celled fungi that are universally present around moisture-laden crops indoors and outdoors; baker's yeast (used for production of carbon dioxide), and brewer's yeast, used for the production of alcohol from sugars

Zeolite: crushed volcanic rock that acts as an effective deodorizer and can be used in shoes as well as the refrigerator. It removes small-molecules such as ammonia, acetone, and smells of mildew from the air and removes heavy metals from water.

Index

About the Author

Born February 9, 1942 in Los Angeles, California, Mark Sneller grew up in Venice/Santa Monica area of Southern California.

He received his Bachelor's Degree in Education from California State Univesity, Los Angeles (1965); Peace Corps India (1965-1967); Master's Degree in Microbiology/Biochemistry, California State University Long Beach; Doctorate from University of Oklahoma in Microbiology/Biochemistry with a specialization in medical mycology (1976); two post-doctoral appointments from the National Institutes of Health in combination drug therapy, and cancer research. Assistant Professor of Microbiology at San Jose State University (1977-1979).

Dr. Sneller began his air quality company, Aero-Allergen Research, in Tucson, Arizona in 1979. He was twice recipient of Clean Air Government Award from the Arizona Lung Association for contributing to better respiratory health of citizens of the state; former member of the State of Arizona Air Pollution Control Hearing Board appointed by the governor; featured in ABC, CBS, NBC national network news, *National Public Radio*; the *New York Times, Newsweek Magazine, Hippocrates Magazine, and Allergic to the 20th Century* (Peter Radetsky, author) for indoor and outdoor air quality work; helped institute and oversaw the nation's first pollen control ordinance; terrorism consultant for City of New York, Department of Human and Mental Services; former contractor with the United States Departments of Justice and Defense; fifteen-year weekly newspaper columnist on air quality; newspaper and television consultant on bioclimatology; fifteen scientific publications in the fields of mycology, fungal toxins, palynology, and incidence of mold around the world; pollen and mold consultant and enumeration expert for the American Academy of Allergy, Asthma and Immunology; radio talk show host for ***The Breathing Easy Show*** (Tucson and Phoenix, Arizona); Sensei with the Japan Karate Association; member of the Society of American Magicians, three-time and current president of the Society of Southwestern Authors.

Other books by Mark R. Sneller: *Time Zone, Cheaters Never Prosper, Dying to Read, The Teleportation Plate, A Breath of Fresh Air.*